Enjoy!

M Fred

Ma 2019

A DAY IN THE LIFE OF A COUNTRY VET

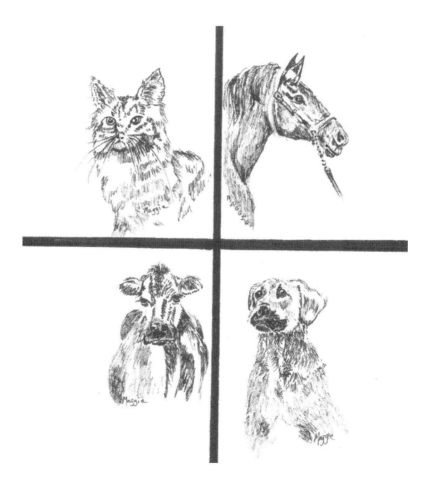

Fred Newschwander DVM

2019

CONTENTS

INTRODUCTION vii

LET'S GO FISHING...1

THE THERAPIST 6

SOLD! 11

DR GRUMPY 16

SOMETHING SHINY 20

JOIN UP!...24

THE GOOD, THE BAD, AND THE UGLY.................................29

THE CAMPING TRIP 39

THE EQUINE EYE 44

HONEYMOON 49

PRACTICING MEDICINE WITHOUT A LICENSE #1 55

$$$$$ 58

PRACTICING MEDICINE WITHOUT A LICENSE #2 62

THE ICELANDIC HORSE..67

ON BEING A STUDENT 71

I WONDER WHERE ALL THE BIRDIES IS 74

THE CUBAN HORSE 76

CUBAN DOGS 81

MY BACKYARD 84

TENNESSEE STUD 90

TOMMY THE BARN CAT 92

16 TONS 94

HISTORIC TRAILS AND ROADS OF KITTITAS COUNTY 100

STAGECOACHES 107

HISTORY OF HORSES IN KITTITAS VALLEY 108

NATURE VS NURTURE 114

BIG LOOP RODEO 118

LAST OF THE KIND 123

GRUMPY OLD MEN 128

MISSING! 136

THE END 141

INTRODUCTION

During my career as a mixed practice veterinarian there were occasional nights when sleep evaded me. Rather than lying there thinking about itches, aches, pains, tomorrow's surgery, or watching the shadows slowly crawl across the ceiling, I sometimes chose to stumble up to my computer and compose stores about people and pets I had encountered during my work. Sometimes I awoke with impressions on my forehead when I fell asleep with my head on the keyboard. In the morning there might be a story in the computer memory worthy of rewriting and editing. Other times it might be gibberish similar to the notes one might make in the middle of the night after waking up from a realistic dream. All too frequently the notes meant nothing and appear to be they work of a raving lunatic finger dancing on the typewriter keyboard.

The better more memorable stories stayed locked away gathering dust in my computer memory until one year I was asked to speak at my 50th university class reunion. I considered talking about how my education prepared me for my career or just cataloging the highlights of my career but the words on the page seemed most uninspiring.

At the last moment I remembered some of my old stories and decided to resurrect and rework them for the presentation. When it was my turn to stand and speak after dinner, I received a brief introduction and proceeded to just read two of my stories. There was some appropriate polite applause and I sat down. The room was pretty quiet as the audience contemplated what I had said and I wondered if I had delivered a total dud. Then the Master of Ceremonies said, "Do you have any more stories?" Thus, I was enthusiastically invited to read another encore story. As the reunion weekend continued classmates and their spouses said, "You ought to write a book." With this encouragement, two years later I completed and self-published "A Day in the Life of a Country Vet."

The writing, editing, formatting and finally publishing proved to be quite a challenge and was also a significant learning process. However, the fire had been lit and the creative juices were flowing albeit somewhat sluggishly. The moderate success of the first book encourage me and six months of attempting to write two to three hours a day resulted in the second book with the original title of "Another Day in the Life of a Country Vet." My slogan and inspiration was the phrase, "A paragraph or two a day hopefully keeps Alzheimer's at bay."

I thought I was out of stories and that my creative well had run dry. In an attempt to keep busy and trying to give something back to my community, I volunteered to do weekly readings of my short stories at senior living and convalescent homes. Additionally, people who had been clients purchased books and often said, "Do you remember when ....? " and I realized there were still many stories as yet untold. The result was this third book in my series which is a little bit of science, some natural history, a little bit of history, a smattering of geography, and more stories about people, their animals, and the relationship between them.

My career inadvertently provided me with the memories and knowledge to have a second very minor career as a writer and publisher. I hope you enjoy this book and the other two as much as I have in writing them. Faites-vous plaisir!

MY DOG PIPER

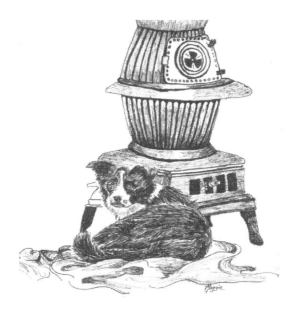

My best friend, footwarmer, trail buddy, alarm clock, dish washer, official assistant/greeter, burglar alarm, telephone ring alerter, muse and proof reader. She also protects against any monsters, sasquatches, or crocodiles that may be lurking under my bed. One of the major drawbacks to owning Border Collies is that they are often more intelligent than their owner.

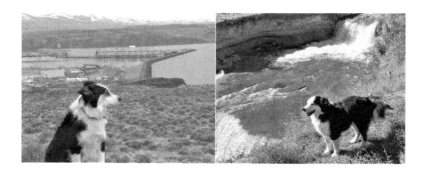

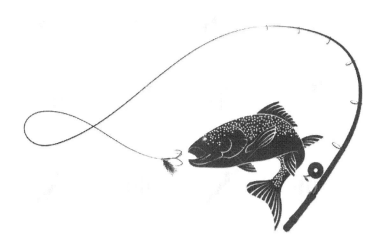

LET'S GO FISHING

In spite of its northern latitude, central Washington is actually located in the Sonoran Desert. If you know where to look, you can find the flattened lobes of yellow flowered Prickly Pear and the barrel shaped red flowered Hedgehog cacti. The area receives only 8 to 10 inches of annual moisture, much of it as snow. It is also home range for two unique western animal species: The Northern Timber Diamondback Rattlesnake and the Westslope Cutthroat Trout. Both species were first described by Meriwether Lewis during the 1804–1806 Lewis and Clark Corps of Discovery expedition. Who would believe that such divergent species would coexist side by side? Snow melt and icy mountain spring waters flow down into the desert canyon landscape where trout can thrive in the riffles and beaver ponds. The grassy/brushy canyon floors walled in by basalt cliffs and rock slides provide an ideal summer and winter habitat for the rattlesnake. I grew near this environment where I hiked, rode my horse, and fished in the streams.

Our family had a wire-haired fox terrier named Susie. We couldn't afford a horse trailer but fortunately we lived in close proximity to the sagebrush covered hills. So, if we wanted to ride our horses in those hills, we first had to travel a few miles on county roads and our dog Susie ran along with us. Once up in the canyons, it was not uncommon to come across a rattlesnake. Rattlesnakes, having really short legs, could sense the ground vibrations as the horses approached, and rather than risk being trampled underfoot, would slither off into the brush or tall grass to get out of the way. If Susie spotted the escape attempt, there was no stopping her. She would grab the snake before it had a chance to coil and kill it by shaking it violently. My sister and I did not think this was particularly remarkable.

The summer I turned 12 or 13 and feeling the need for an adventure, I had the bright idea of going fishing in one of these canyons. Umtanum Creek Canyon flows from west to east down a thrust fold fault line in Umtanum Ridge. The north wall of the canyon has many basalt rock slides which are a great winter denning environment for rattlesnakes. The valley floor is full of willows and alders which provide food for beavers and cover for small rodents otherwise known as snake food.

I decided to take my zero-horsepower steed known as Schwinn. I tied the laces of my irrigating boots together and threw them over the handlebars and I taped my fishing pole to the frame. A small backpack contained some snacks, P&J sandwich, and some other fishing gear. I dug a few worms, caught a few grasshoppers, and checked to be sure that there was still some "Soft but Satisfying" fish egg bait in the Pautzke's jar.

It was about six hilly miles to Umtanum Creek but the weather was pleasant and there was a warm sun in my face. The road passed by the Damman school house, part of which was constructed in 1893. It was, of course, closed for the summer but the chain swings swayed languidly in the light summer breeze. From there the road turned to gravel and worked its way up into the mouth of Shushuskin Canyon named after a Native American who lived there in the mid-1800s. By standing on the pedals and pumping, I could climb most of the grade but when the washboard got too bad, I had to get off and push. My eagerness to go fishing began to wane. Some quail flushed from the roadside brush and disappeared off into a side canyon and a red tail hawk screeched from above perhaps annoyed that I had alerted his potential dinner. The road finally reached the top of the canyon where the Durr Road branched left and to the southeast. As it traversed the top of North Umtanum Ridge it skirted the rolling winter wheat fields that you could smell maturing in the midsummer heat. From there the two-track range road dropped into a small canyon and with the bicycle chain clattering against the frame I eventually switch backed to the valley floor of Umtanum Creek. When the Durr road was built in 1882 and it was a toll route providing a shortcut between Ellensburg and the Wenas Valley. Big wide sweeping switch back corners were built into the road so that the six-in-hand freight pulling horse teams could negotiate them. The leaders, the pair in the front of the hitch, had to side step around these great arcs so the wagon could clear the inside corner.

When I finally arrived at the ford where the road crossed the creek, I was tired, sweaty, and my fingers were numb from clutching the vibrating bicycle handlebars but I couldn't wait to begin fishing. The heavy smell of sage tickled my nose but I hurriedly assembled my pole and tackle and put a sticky stinky salmon egg on the hook. After pulling on my rubber irrigating boots, I pushed through the brush and worked my way up stream while a small covey of chuckers darted up the hillside in front of me. It wasn't long before I caught my first bright 8-inch cutthroat trout. I laughed out loud at the fun I was having but there was no one else to laugh with me. I felt a momentary pang of loneliness.

A desert sagebrush lined canyon stream seemed an unusual place to find a mountain trout. I soon had a half a dozen small trout and I suddenly realized that I was famished. Who would have guessed that fishing could be such hard work? I scrambled back down the stream bank to my bicycle and found my brown bag waiting. We drank creek water in those days so after splashing off my sweaty face and lying belly down to get a cold drink, I sat on a fallen down cottonwood log and I opened my sack lunch. It didn't take long to eat my P & J, peel and eat my orange, and inhale my mother's homemade raisin cookies. It's amazing that whatever flavor or type of sandwich you start out with, by the time you carry it around all day, it always turns into a squashed field mouse sandwich. Life was good but I suspect a 12 or 13-year-old didn't fully appreciate that.

I almost fell asleep sitting there in the afternoon sun but I finally roused myself and pivoted around on my fanny putting my right foot down on the other side of the log. I was startled when something thumped my right rubber boot at ankle level. I looked and was shocked to see a 3-foot rattlesnake already coiling back up again. Fancy meeting him there! He must have been there the whole time also taking a nap in the warm mid-day sun. Obviously, I politely retreated to my side of the log and waited at least 5 minutes for my heart to return to my chest and commence beating again. My boots had protected me from the snake fangs but I still pulled my boot off to make sure that I needn't anticipate imminent death. When I looked back over the log, my new friend Mr. N. T. D. Rattlesnake was slithering off to disappear into the grass and brush. I don't know if I stepped on him or just came very close, but obviously he objected to my lack of respect for his personal space.

They air suddenly felt chill as if a cloud had passed in front of the sun and I felt very much alone. Easily convincing myself that I had enough fish, I decided that I would end my fishing excursion and hurry home. I pedaled my trusty Schwinn back up the switchbacks, past the wheat fields, but enjoyed the thrill of coasting down the long grade back to the Damman School House. When I got home, I wanted to tell someone what had happened but decided that my mother would survive just fine not knowing the finer details of my fishing adventure.

I now know that the Northern Timber Diamondback Rattlesnake is the least aggressive and the least venomous of the Crotalus genus. On many occasions I have cautiously escorted them with a long stick to get off trails or out of roadways where they were sunning themselves trying to convince them that these were not good places to sleep. A gasoline consuming internal combustion machine or some Macho he-man was likely to come along to cause their untimely demise.

Rattlesnakes hunt by ambush. Small rodents leave pheromone trails where they habitually travel that the snake can *smell* with its forked tongue. When the rodent passes by they strike and envenomate it. They wait a few minutes until the rodent has expired and then follow the trail to enjoy their warm fresh meal in a leisurely uninterrupted fashion.

Cutthroat trout are much more dangerous, that is if you are some sort of an insect or worm. However, it pays to be cautious if wading barefoot in a trout stream. You might discover when you sit to put on your shoes and socks that a trout has stolen some of your toes when you weren't paying attention

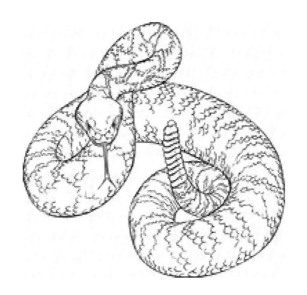

Mr. N T D Rattlesnake, Esq

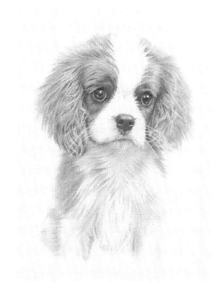

THE THERAPIST

Dr. Mike was our family physician. He was also our friend. He practiced during an era with less specialization and thus performed almost all medical procedures. He did our vaccinations, gave us our physicals, stitched up my face after a serious dog bite, administered our pregnancy test, provided prenatal checkups, and delivered our son. We socialized with his family, played racket sports, and I ski patrolled with him in the winter at a nearby ski resort.

When it came time for my vasectomy, he was more than glad to oblige. "Anything for a friend," he said with a slightly evil grin. We took care of that minor little medical procedure late one Friday afternoon after he had finished his office appointments.

"Would you mind if two of my medical interns observed"? he asked.

What could I say? After all we were both medical professionals and it seemed appropriate to help in the education of future practitioners. Too late I realized that I had fallen into his trap when he introduced Dr. Sally Brown and Dr. Georgia Smith. When I caught his eye, he couldn't help but display a little smirk.

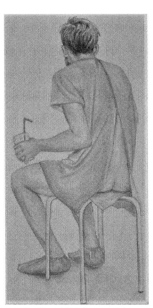

Snip, snip, stitch, stitch and it was all over.

The next day we attended a dinner party at his house. He clinked his drink glass with a spoon to get everyone's attention and announced, "I would like to introduce the newest member of our local Soprano Boys Choir: Dr Fred." I eventually got somewhat even with him when I paid him 2 cords of firewood for his surgical services. I didn't own any chickens or ducks.

It was a fairly small community and it was only reasonable that we would have some clients in common. He would see the two-legged members of a family and I might attend to the four-legged members. HIPAA rules were not formerly established at that time so it was not uncommon for Dr. Mike and I to discretely compare notes and discuss cases. He might say that, "Mrs. Smith has some sort of a rash that I can't diagnose."

I might respond by asking, "Does she sleep with her cat"? Problem solved! Mrs. Smith was being bitten by the fleas that had set up housekeeping on her cat. There were times when I benefited from his more extensive knowledge of internal medicine issues. It was a friendly symbiotic medical relationship.

Late on a Friday winter evening Dr. Mike called just as I was leaving my office. The weather was cold and bleak and you could see the sleet bouncing off the pavement. I wasn't particularly eager to step outside and get blasted by the weather, so I walked back inside and settled into my soft warm office nap chair. Mike asked, "Have you got a minute"?

I said, "Sure. My wife and son are out of town to visit her family for the weekend and I'm on call so I've got all night."

He said, "In that case, why don't we meet for a beer"?

We settled back in a booth at a local pub and quickly finished off a bowl of beer nuts and a brew. I asked, "Didn't you have some sort of a question for me"?

Dr. Mike said, "It felt so good to get off my feet and relax I almost forgot. I have a client, Joan .... who has had a fairly serious stroke. She's recovering nicely but may never be able to totally take care of herself. She doesn't have any family to assist so she decided that she should move into an extended care facility. The problem is, she has a dog. She's walking a little and talking pretty well now and told me that you were her dog's veterinarian. She's pretty worried about her dog. Do you have any idea what we can do with it?"

I asked, "Can't she take the dog with her to the nursing home"?

Mike replied, "I talked to the administrator and she said, 'Absolutely not. It would be disruptive and the dog might carry diseases.'"

I said, "That's total nonsense," but as I recall I used somewhat spicier language. I said, "I'll go talk to the administrator and see what we can do."

We finished our beer and emptied the second bowl of beer nuts and walked out into the cold and 2 inches of new wet sloppy snow.

On Monday morning I called the nursing home and introduced myself and explained what I wanted to discuss. We set up an appointment with the administrator for late that afternoon. When I walked into her office and introduced myself, the look on her face was not encouraging. She attempted a friendly smile but her jaw was firmly set and she had that determined look in her eye. I think she already had the relevant information but I again explained how the only friend this woman had was Prince Charlie, her King Charles Cavalier Spaniel. I think I got a somewhat sympathetic response but she went on to explain that the health and welfare of the rest of the residents had to take precedence. I thanked her for her time and went home to contemplate any other options. In the meantime, my staff and I took turns taking the delightful Prince Charlie home with us at night.

About a week later I tried again. When I spoke to the administrator, I said, "I am willing to vouch for the health of the dog and will make sure it is vaccinated, bathed, and well-groomed. Can't we at least bring it in for short visits during the quiet times between meals. We will be certain to not be disruptive."

The only response I got was, "Well, we'll think about it."

A few days later I tried again through a telephone call. I think I was beginning to wear her down because she said, "OK. We'll give it one try."

We set up a time to bring Prince Charlie in during the afternoon when most of the residents would be taking their afternoon nap and the facility would be pretty quiet. We brushed Prince Charlie's teeth, cleaned his ears, trimmed and filed his toenails, give him a bath and blow dry, and put a pretty blue ribbon in his top knot.

I was met officiously in the lobby by the administrator who personally escorted me down the hall to room #17. When I entered the room, Joan was asleep and it took a moment for her to wake up and recognize me. We chatted for a few moments and then she heard very quiet little yips and whines down at floor level. The expression on her face changed from quiet resignation to pure ecstatic joy. Unassisted, she managed to get off her bed and collapse on the floor where an ecstatic emotional reunion occurred. The sniffing of tears, sobs of joy, and quiet little yips were the only sounds in the room.

After 15 minutes, the administrator, who I suspect had been lurking out in the hallway the whole time, returned and said, "It's time for Prince Charlie to go home now."

Not wanting to rock the boat, Prince Charlie and I complied but as we were escorted down the hall I said, "Can we come back next week?"

The expression on her face indicated reluctance but nevertheless she said, "I suppose!" That routine continued twice a week for several weeks but our visiting time gradually extended from 15 minutes to half an hour and then to an hour. The word got out and many of the other residents, pushing their walkers in front of them, or driving their wheel chairs begin showing up in

Joan's room during that visitation period. The administrator looked on with an expression of disapproval but nevertheless showed self-control and didn't say anything.

A few weeks later I took a calculated high-risk gamble. About halfway through the visit I accidentally on purpose unclipped Prince Charlie's leash and turned him loose. He seemed to know where all the rooms were for the residents who had come to visit him in Joan's room and he quietly traveled down the hall from room to room to say hello to them all. The administrator couldn't help herself and had to smile when she saw what was happening. The next step was an all-day visit followed by and overnight sleep over. Eventually my devious plan succeeded and when I asked her, she agreed to allow extended stays. Eventually, Prince Charlie became a permanent unpaid resident therapist of the nursing home facility. The staff happily volunteered to take turns being Prince Charlie's escort and guardian for a day and to take him outside frequently for exercise and potty breaks. At night he slept in his own special bed at the foot of Joan's bed. Eventually she improved to the point where, with her walker, she could take Prince Charlie outside herself. I made frequent visits to check on him and hold up my end of the bargain to ensure that he was always clean and posed no health risk to any of the residents. A few months later when I came to check on Charlie, I listened and was sure I heard the distinctive sound of a small dog barking. I eased down the hall and peered into a room to see a sweet little long-haired Chihuahua named Chewy doing the Cha-Cha on his owner's bed. During subsequent conversations with the administrator she said, "I came to realize the residents were much more active and engaged with pets in the facility and any risk was far outweighed by the positive impact."

The Fair Housing Act of 1973 started the legal process of allowing animals into public housing and it was further refined in 2013 to include virtually all assistance animals.

Joan quietly passed in her sleep a few years later but Prince Charlie continued his mental and physical therapy sessions until he too succumbed to the inevitable ravages of old age. His legacy is that he opened the doors in that facility to a continuum of other four-legged therapists

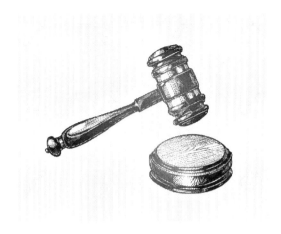

SOLD!

As the human mind and body age, limitations in attitude and activity level are sometimes required. A younger person might prefer a four-wheel drive truck or a powerful sports car. With the approach of middle age transportation preferences might drift towards Cadillacs and Camrys. Such can be the case with equestrians.

One day my wife and I discovered that we had suddenly become middle aged. What a surprise! Where did our youth go? Perhaps powerful quarter horses might not be the perfect choice for a mount. Something quieter and smoother might be more appropriate. When we lost a special quarter horse mare to blindness, we looked around for another breed alternative. A knowledgeable local horseman encouraged us to consider Tennessee Walker horses. We looked around locally and on the west side of the Cascade Mountains and tried out some horses but couldn't find what we wanted.

We eventually wound up in Spokane at Reinbeau Ranches and purchased our first quality Tennessee Walking Horse. We discovered that Janet, the owner, was very knowledgeable about the breed, the bloodlines, and the trainers in Tennessee and she traveled east several times a year to purchase horses. These were horses that had extensive training but perhaps weren't quite fancy enough for the show ring or had progressed as far as they could in the show circuit.

I asked Janet if she ever needed assistance bringing horses from Shelbyville, Tennessee back to Spokane, Washington. She quickly replied, "Would you? I would love to have some help. I buy 14 horses and trailer them back to Spokane. It's a pretty grueling adventure."

The Celebration is the largest Tennessee Walker horse show and happens in late August of every year. There is arena show competition and in conjunction with that are several horse sales. We arranged to fly out to Nashville while she drove her horse hauler from Spokane. We met her there to assist as she purchased and collected horses. We would then help her drive cross-country back to Spokane.

One afternoon we had to shelter under the Celebration show ring grandstands while a massive thunderstorm parked overhead. The show resumed after dark an hour later and we watched the best Tennessee Walkers in the world strut their stuff. The next two days we attended the horse sales to find horses that could be repurposed as pleasure horses in the Pacific Northwest.

At one sale there was a magnificent trained stallion for sale and the bidding had not reached appropriate levels. So, the auctioneer temporarily but melodramatically paused the auction and asked, "Is there anybody in the audience who wants to ride this spectacular horse?"

Of course, the auctioneer had prearranged for someone qualified and prepared to be in attendance should such an occasion arise. The bidding improved somewhat but was still not as high as the quality the horse might indicate.

The auctioneer asked, "Does anyone *else* want to ride this wonderful stallion?"

My wife, encouraged by Janet, raised her hand. She had never ridden a show quality Tennessee Walker and required a little coaching to allow the horse to fully demonstrate its gaits. Ultimately, because of this ride by an inexperienced rider, the horse sold for an additional $1,500.

We were just there to observe and help and were having a great experience. During a break, I went off to the little boy's room and to get soft drinks. When I came back, my wife had her hand in air bidding on a horse. This was not something we had discussed or planned for and I was obviously more than a little surprised.

This was during the recession of 2008 and horse prices were unusually low. Additionally, there was a drought in the Tennessee Walker breeding country of southeastern United States, so pasture was short and breeders we're having to unload horses. Horses that should have sold for $3000 to $5,000 and up were selling for $1,000. So, I diplomatically held my tongue and we became the proud owner of a new horse. I discussed the issue more with Janet and she convinced me that most of these horses could be retrained and sold for profit out west in Washington State. Not wanting to be outdone by my wife, I bought a young gelding also, deciding that I needed a project horse. But does a wise horseman (or veterinarian) purchase an unexamined horse only after seeing it pass back and forth on the runway of a sales barn? Needless to say, I felt pretty vulnerable and had to rely on Janet's knowledge of horse bloodlines and skill of the trainers. Thus, we bought two horses never having ridden them, picked up their feet, worked around them, or done any kind of a health check.

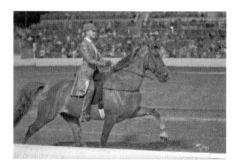

Eventually we had 2 horses and Janet had 12 and at 2 AM, to avoid the commuter traffic gridlock around Nashville and the nasty torrid temperatures and humidity, we started our drive westward. It was **Wagons Ho!** Janet had done this many time before and had arrangements at livestock sales yards in Sioux Falls and Butte where she could stop and rest the horses for a few hours overnight. She would just put a check in an envelope and put it in the icebox in the feed room. At daylight we would reload the horses and continued driving. When we stopped at rest areas to give ourselves and the horses a break, we opened all the windows on the trailer to let the horses stick their heads out. In no time at all we had crowds of traveling families with kids gathered around who wanted to pet the horses. We knew some of the horses well enough by then to know that they were safe and so standing cautiously nearby, let mothers lift their children up to meet and pet their first ever horse.

We finally arrived home with two horses of unknown quality. Over time, we got to know and love them and appreciate their personalities, training, and steadiness. They were willing learners and easily adapted to their new circumstances. I suspect that the horse I purchased and never really been out of the barn or allowed to run free in a pasture. It took him a while to learn how to follow a trail. Some two months later I happened to look into the mouth of the mare my wife I purchased. There had been no opportunity to examine her except from a distance in Tennessee. I was shocked to discover that she was missing her upper front incisors. Horses can be born without permanent teeth buds and that appeared to be the case with Morticia. Her missing teeth have never been a problem and she grazes and chews as well as any horse that has a full set of teeth.

Subsequently, my wife discovered that she liked another gelding more than the mare she had purchased. This is how I came to own a tall leggy Sabino Tennessee Walking mare with a bold blaze down her nose but lacking two front teeth. I guess that's why she had fit right into hillbilly country of Tennessee.

Morticia has been part of my life now for 10 years and must be 22 years old now. She has learned to love mountain trails and willingly does anything I ask of her. When trail terrain allows, she can shift into a running walk and can travel up to 20 miles an hour. I don't think it is possible for a rider to encourage a Tennessee Walker horse and ride this fast smooth gait without a smile on their face. At 22 years of age she would have to be considered an elderly lady but is showing no signs of slowing down. I suspect she may be the last horse of my riding career.

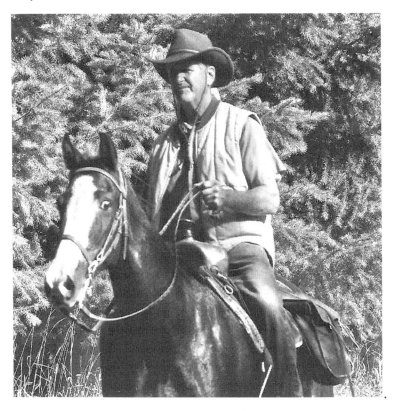

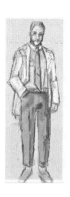

DR GRUMPY

In November of 1889 Washington became a state. Four months later in March of 1890 the federal land grant institution called the State Agricultural College and School of Science was established by the state legislature. Soon after it was renamed Washington State College and in 1957 it became Washington State University which now has an enrollment of over 29,000 students. In 1899 the School of Veterinary Science was established with one professor and three students. Present class size is about 125 students per class (500 total) with 60 faculty members.

At that time Pullman was a logical location for a college because it was in the center of the Palouse agricultural area. Farming was mainly horse powered so establishing a college of veterinary science there made logical sense. Subsequently, the main population centers of the state are 200 miles away west of the Cascades and farming is mainly accomplished by internal combustion machine. The Washington State University College of Veterinary Medicine is a fine multimillion-dollar Institution. However, one of its shortcomings is insufficient patient and client load since it is so far removed from major population centers and thus their animals and pets. There is a shortage of routine medical and surgical issues from which the students could gain valuable exposure and training.

In the 1960's and 70's, many of the animals presented at the school were referrals from elsewhere in the state. They might have been complex cases requiring the surgery skills, diagnostic expertise, or specialized facilities of the veterinary school and faculty. On occasion the cost of treating an animal could exceed a client's ability to pay. In that era one way to enhance the experience for the students was to have the animal donated to the school. The school covered the cost of treatment in trade for ownership and an enhanced student learning opportunity. Many of these animals were eventually returned to the original owner or adopted by one of the veterinary students.

One such animal was Sammy. He weighed about 25 lb., had one erect ear and one floppy ear, wore a medium length blonde curly hair coat, and had a long tail that seemed to have a mind of its own. His ancestry was ... mixed. He came from somewhere north of Seattle and was referred by his local veterinarian who couldn't come up with a diagnosis or treatment for his chronic cough. Sammy's human siblings had grown up and left the nest. His parents liked to travel and felt a little burdened by Sammy. He had thus been donated to the veterinary school. I could never quite comprehend why such a delightful little dog would be abandoned but such was his plight.

Part of learning the science and the art of veterinary medicine is memorizing lists of possible causes for ailments or complaints. Real life doesn't always follow the text books however. Every veterinarian who has worked with dogs has had clients come in saying that their dog must have gotten something such as a fishbone caught in its throat and this is why the animal is coughing. But I know of very few veterinarians who have ever diagnosed such an event. Why can't medical issues follow the rules?

Sammy actually had a history of exposure to small steak bones. When an x-ray revealed nothing in his throat or digestive system to indicate a bone, it was assumed he had kennel cough, a disease caused by a combination of a virus and bacteria, and was sent home to recover. But after several weeks he was still not particularly sick but had frequent coughing bouts especially after drinking or eating wet food.

Even testing at the veterinary school did not reveal a cause but he was such a sweet little dog that he was kept around for the students to study. He was well cared for and taken for frequent walks but excitement or activity always seemed to prompt a coughing bout. Students rotated through different clinic sections at about 1-month intervals.

When I was assigned to the internal medicine ward, Sammy became my patient. He had been there so long that everyone had lost interest in his case and felt all avenues of investigation had been explored. Being only a student, I did not know that dogs never got bones caught in their throat. I surmised that if Sammy had swallowed a small bone and it got stuck in his throat for several days it could puncture a hole from the esophagus to the trachea. We call this a tracheal esophageal fistula. Obviously, if Sammy consumed a liquid it could leak through this hole into his airways and cause coughing. But the professor in charge didn't want to listen to the incoherent ramblings of a student. He was known to all the students as being especially grumpy and a difficult task master particularly when he was instructing students in his surgery lab. No one liked to butt heads with him.

Knowing that I was unlikely to change his mind I looked elsewhere for help. There was a professor in radiology who was a fairly recent addition to the faculty and was not too far removed from having a student himself. He was not grumpy and was known for being willing to help students.

I spoke to him and he said, "I would be glad to help but we'll have to do it when Dr Grumpy is not around."

My theory was that there was a fistula or tunnel which would allow liquid to escape from the esophagus into the trachea and airways. My plan was to have him swallow barium, a liquid medium that would show up on an x-ray, to see if any of it leaked and showed up in the lungs. Lo and behold, it did and produced what we would call a classical air bronchogram because some of the barium dispersed into the lung fields.

When I took this evidence to Dr Grumpy, he said, "Well, you must have administered it to him too fast!"

So, I approached Dr Friendly again and with his assistance we administered barium with a feeding tube that bypassed his oropharynx (the swallowing area) thus eliminating the possibility of drowning him if I gave him the barium too fast. Again, we got an air bronchogram which was consistent with a more distant connection between the esophagus and the trachea. Dr. Grumpy was still not impressed with my evidence. About that time, we went through our clinical rotations and I moved on to another section leaving Sammy to his fate

One of my classmates inherited Sammy's case and she approached me one day during lunch hour. She said, "I hear you butted heads with Dr Grumpy."

I laughed and said, "I guess I did."

She went on to explain how he had discussed Sammy's case with her section of students and how he had personally ruled out a tracheal esophageal fistula.

Sammy had been our guest for about six months and most of my class had taken a look at him but nobody wanted to question Dr Grumpy. My classmate, Shirley, who it inherited his case, had finally been assigned the distressing task of euthanizing him since his usefulness had diminished and we had still not been able to diagnosis the reason for his cough.

Every day in vet school brings new challenges and learning opportunities so, being occupied elsewhere, I more less forgot about Sammy. Occasionally his smiling face and wagging tail would come to mind.

One day about a month later I happen to encounter Dr Grumpy as we passed in the hallway. He said, "If you have a minute could you stop in to my office"?

I said, "I have a break before my next class so now would be perfect." I sat down on an uncomfortable wooden chair in his office while he searched through a folder on his desk.

He said, "I just got this postmortem pathology report and thought you would like to see it." There was a pained look on his face but I couldn't interpret just what it meant. After I read the brief report and put it back down on his desk he said, "You were right! Dammit! I guess there's an important lesson here for both of us. First of all, you were correct. It appears the sharp point of a bone penetrated the wall of the esophagus and caused a tracheal esophageal fistula. It would have been a very complicated open chest surgery to repair, but it could have been done. Secondly, this case emphasizes the importance of being good listener; for me and for you as you prepare for a career as a practicing veterinarian. Thirdly, if you go into a situation with a preconceived notion for the outcome, you decrease the chances of reaching the correct conclusion."

Dr. Grumpy, in a very rare moment of humility and contrition said, "I liked Sammy too and deeply regret that I made the erroneous decision to have him euthanized." He then stood up and said, "That'll be all."

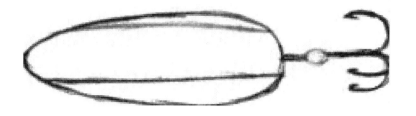

SOMETHING SHINY

It was going to be a hot Saturday afternoon; probably up into the mid-nineties. It was perhaps too hot for a ride but had it been too long since I'd had a break from work. We discussed our options and decided that after my last morning appointment we would trailer the horses up into the mountains where the temperature would be more comfortable. We were already sweaty and dirty by the time we got the horses and our dog Liz loaded. She was not very heat tolerant so we made sure we had plenty of water in the saddle bags and had chosen a route with frequent watering holes and stream crossings. On these adventures, like Superman in his phone booth, she frequently made the transition from a moderately well-groomed apricot poodle to the very rare breed of black-footed poodle. How black footed depended on the color and consistency of the mud she used to cool down.

The road up Manastash Canyon was dry and dusty and not having been graded for some time, the washboards were well established and waiting for us. I'm not sure why they are called washboards because you weren't particularly clean after using them. When we unloaded at the trailhead for Shoestring Lake, I began to wonder about the wisdom of our choice. Even the birds were quiet in the mid-day heat but we were committed and decided to forge ahead anyway.

Just before we left my wife inquired, "Are there any fish up there?"

I replied, "There used to be some nice cutthroat but I haven't been there for quite a few years."

As an afterthought I got some fishing tackle out of the truck and put it in my saddlebags. My wife loved to fish but didn't really like to eat them. Consequently, most of our fishing was catch-and-release and we carefully returned most of them to their water world unless they were hurt. In that case, the fish volunteered to come home with us for dinner to join in an impromptu fish barbeque.

The horses powered up the trail and needed a little encouragement because they weren't particularly enjoying the hard work or sweaty dripping bodies. Fortunately, the trail passed into virgin old growth timber along a stream and it felt like the temperature must have dropped 15 degrees. We stopped beside a large quiet pool to cool off and let everybody have a drink. The higher we climbed the more pleasant it got and the more our attitude improved. The mountain air was rejuvenating and the birds were singing again.

We eventually rode through a gap in the trees and there before us was Shoestring Lake. It was a small narrow ribbon of a lake fed by a spring that at bubbled out from the toe of a basalt rock slide. The lake was like a mirror and reflected perfect images of the canyon walls, Lodgepole Pines, and Alpine firs. Even the faint full moon in the mid-day sky could be seen in the mirrored reflection. The scene was deserted and there was no sign that anyone had even recently been there. We dismounted, loosened the girth on the horses, and give them a long drink in the cold waters of the lake. After getting a drink ourselves, we found a log in the sun and sat to eat our sandwiches and snack on some Oreo cookies.

Then we heard a faint splash behind us in the lake. We both turned to see the widening ripples left by a cutthroat trout jumping after a bug on the glassy lake surface. My wife could hardly contain her excitement, so I got the fishing pole assembled and attached the reel. More fish were jumping as I fed the line down through the guides. I returned to the saddle bag to look for the lures. I dumped the contents on the ground to be struck with the realization that they were still down in the truck. Somebody (me) had forgotten to put some in the saddlebags.

Boy! Was I ever in trouble! There was an obvious look of disappointment on my wife's face but she refrained from commenting on how disorganized her husband was. The fish were really jumping now, probably feeding on a mayfly hatch. Fortunately, we had a few Oreo cookies left but there was no Budweiser beer. Dejectedly, we sat on the gravely bank of the lake and watched fish swimming at our feet and jumping further out on the lake. In the crystal-clear water, however, I noticed something flashing faintly some distance out from the shore.

I said to my wife, "It looks like somebody has been fishing here and got snagged and lost some lures out on the bottom."

The temperature was pleasant so I found a grassy spot in the sun to take a short practice nap. Sometime later I was awakened by the sound of splashing. It must have been a giant fish. I sat up to see my wife striped down to her underwear diving to retrieve the lures from the lake bottom. I stumbled over to bravely stand on the lake shore and pretend to assist her as she clambered up out of the lake. She had almost turned blue, her teeth were chattering, and she was totally covered in goosebumps, but she had a huge smile on her face. I thought I heard a Steller's Jay squawking derisively in some nearby branches. Was a buck deer spying at my exposed wife? After we got her dried off with an old sweatshirt, and dressed back in her Levi's and shirt, we examined her treasure trove. There were three sets of fishing lures each in a different state of disassembly and disrepair.

We salvaged and polished a little spinner, repurposed some lead split shot, rethreaded some orange plastic beads, and managed to salvage 1/3 of a treble hook with one semi sharp point remaining. We found a piece of sandstone and sharpened the hook.

The smile returned to my wife's face when she cast out in the lake and hooked a nice fat cutthroat trout on her first attempt. It appeared that I would be forgiven. It was perfect for her because the hook had no barb and once she got the fish reeled in close to the shore, she could ease the tension on the line and the fish could wiggle off to, *Swim away and catch some bugs another day*.

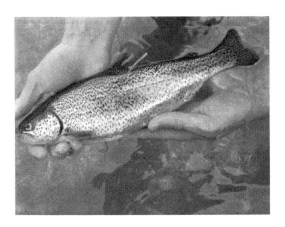

One fish was slightly injured and there was some uncertainty as to whether it would survive. So, we gathered a few small twigs and started a tiny fire in some moist dirt near the lake shore. We skewered the unfortunate volunteer on a green stick and toasted it over the fire until the flesh started curling away from the bones. Even my wife had to admit it was pretty tasty.

"I don't think I ever had to work so hard to get my dinner," she said. The perfect conclusion to our adventure came when a camp robber (also known as a grey jay or whiskey jack) landed on my wife's outstretched hand to steal bits of bread crust. Evening was approaching so we readied our horses and rode down out of the mountains to our waiting horse trailer. The road didn't seem quite so dusty and rough on the trip out. Perhaps our attitude had been changed because of the delightful afternoon spent at Shoestring Lake.

Soon it would be Monday morning and time to begin another busy work week.

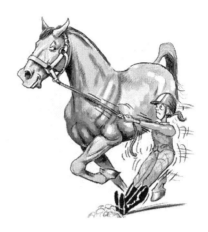

JOIN UP!

In the cowboy tradition of the American west, harsh methods involving pain and fear were sometimes used to train horses. There was a need to rapidly break large numbers semi-feral horses to meet the economic demands of the expanding west.

With the advent of the internal combustion engine, horse numbers and use rapidly declined and they were much more likely to be used for pleasure rather than industry. When the horse became our friend rather than our tool, more humane techniques came into play. In the 1980's the concept of modern natural horsemanship techniques as practiced by legendary horsemen Tom Dorrance, Ray Hunt, Buck Brannaman, and Pat Parelli were quantified and gained popular acceptance. One of the tenants is the application of gentle physical pressure which is released when the horse complies or *pressure and release*. Their work was portrayed, with some significant inaccuracies, in Robert Redford's popular film "The Horse Whisperer".

Monty Roberts first published horse training books in 1996 and released his book "Horse Sense for People" in the year 2002. Too bad it wasn't released 50 years earlier when I could have used it. The book documents Monty's training techniques and his philosophy regarding animals. His work may have been inspired by or at least partially parallels the earlier work of his predecessors.

Here's the scene: I'm 7 years old and my sister is 10. She can still beat up on me and run faster. It's summertime, school is out, and the city swimming pool is open if you can get there. But we live in rural Kittitas County 5 miles out of town, there are no other kids our age in the neighborhood, and our family only has one car. Our father is a chemistry professor but this is not a career noted for great financial reward. Consequently, during the summer, he supplements the family income teaching university summer school classes or by doing chemical analysis for a local food processing company. We have no TV, no Gameboys, no cell phones, no fast food, and life is pretty tough. We did not realize it until 10 years later but our mother is a school teacher who has MS and spends much of her time just feeling tired or recovering from being tired

They were good parents but they were pretty occupied just getting through life, so, we were left to our own devices to keep ourselves entertained. If we got bored, we only had ourselves to blame. Often, after we got our house, yard, and garden chores done, we might decide to go for a ride on the horses.

We only had one saddle so I typically got the unique privilege of riding bareback. We would pull the halters off their hooks in the leather smelling tack room and fill a bucket with grain from the bin and walk out into the five-acre pasture to catch the horses. They would typically hurry up for the grain but once they got a mouthful they would duck away before we could get a halter on them.

And then the game, for the horses at least, began. They would circle around us staying just out of reach and typically eventually gallop away. They quickly discerned who the targets were and typically used the unwanted horses to hide behind. Dragging the bucket and halter ropes behind us, we would dutifully follow after them only to repeat the same drama at the other end of the pasture. Our failure led to frustration and soon the horses were galloping merrily around the field with us running after. Eventually we spilled all the grain, threw the empty halters and even heaved horse road apples at them as well. At least there was no shortage of ammunition to throw. After we trooped from one end of the pasture to the other half a dozen times, the situation exceeded the frustration capacity of two pre-teen equestrians. Yelling in frustration accomplished nothing accept the possibility of children walking back to the barn with tears streaming down their faces. That seemed to be the signal for the horses to begin acting like well trained horses rather than uncatchable four-legged demons whose only goal was to torment us. The horses would eventually stop and turn until they were facing us. If we stood where we were, they might eventually even walk a few steps closer to us. At that point if we could still find the halters, we could walk up to the horses, put the halters on, and lead them to the barn. It was a game for the horses but that was certainly not a fun game for two small children. At that age we had no understanding of horse behavior and only knew that eventually we had succeeded in catching our horse. At least we were finally able to fulfill our plan of going for a horseback ride in the nearby sage covered hills.

Sometimes you felt that horses could read your mind. Actually, they probably were reading our body language. If you went out to the barn to feed them, they were willing participants in the activity. Somehow your body must have looked different if you walked out to the barn intending to catch and ride the horses because then they became very difficult to catch.

20 years later I had become veterinarian and had to treat and work with horses on a fairly regular basis. Sometimes the horse was kept at a place remote from the owner's residence and so they might say "I'll just meet you out at the pasture."

This often started mental alarm bells ringing because inevitably when we got to the pasture, the horses had not been caught and my presence only seem to exacerbate the situation. Sometimes we had to give up catching the horse and reschedule. Reluctantly, I had to say, "I'm sorry but I'm just too busy today to be a horse wrangler."

On some occasions, if we had three or four people, we would just keep the horses moving around and around the field until they finally gave up and we were able to catch them. You knew you were close to success if a horse dropped its head and licked its lips and chewed as it circled around you. I assumed in those days that the horses finally got tired and just decided to let us win.

As time went on, I refined my technique and learned to position people around a pasture and the goal was to just keep the horses moving. If they slowed down to a walk or stopped, we would encourage them to keep moving again and circle around us. I must admit I never examined the issue from the point of view of horse training techniques and their instinctive response to the situation. At least I didn't have to throw manure clods, halters, buckets, and shed any tears if I had to walk forlornly back to my truck.

Finally, in the year 2002 I had an answer or explanation as to what had been going on. Monty Roberts used and popularized the phrase "Joining up." He and other horse whispers could take an unbroken horse into a round pen and start it circling. They explained that if you stepped slightly behind line of sight of the horse and in line with his rump the horse would circle forward. If you stepped slightly in front of the horse more in line with his eyes, a horse would slow, stop, or pivot and go in the opposite direction. If you keep the horse going around long enough, but not to the point of showing stress or exhaustion, eventually he would drop his head with his muzzle closer to the ground and might begin licking his lips and demonstrate a chewing action. Soon the horse would likely stop, turn towards you, and even take a few steps in your direction. This is what Monty Roberts called *Joining Up*. Early proponents of the technique might use noises or whips or relatively unpleasant means to startle a horse and keep it circling. In a sense that was what I had been doing in large open horse pastures accept my round pen was 5 acres or more and not only 75 feet in diameter.

Contemporary horse behavioralists have studied this more deeply and use the term *Pressure and release*. Mild pressure is applied to the horse in a round pen or enclosure to keep the horse moving. The trainer steps back from the horse thus releasing the pressure. Eventually the horse realizes that if it stops and turns towards the trainer the pressure will be released. This is one of the basic tenants of equine training. More recently, *Joining Up* has been explained by saying that gentle pressure applied to the horse stimulates a nervous system response resulting in increased salivation. The results are licking, chewing, and swallowing. Fortunately, horses have never learned to spit like a cowboy.

It had been previously thought that the trainer was mimicking the actions of a dominant horse, like a herd stallion or lead mare, chasing a young colt away from the herd. It was felt that the horse would eventually submit in an attempt to be allowed to rejoin or *Join Up* with the herd. Further experimentation has shown that

27

mimicking a horse is not at all essential. Researchers have even used very small toy remote battery cars to quietly chase horse in a round pen situation. When the car backs away, the horse stops, turns, and often even curiously approaches the car. Thus, pressure applied and then released, can be used to train the horse. If the trainer can communicate to the horse what he wants and then apply quiet pressure and then release it if the horse responds appropriately, a lesson can be learned.

It's interesting to note that a horse in a new or unusual environment might seem easier to catch. If they are well trained, they seem to sense the pressure of the situation and know that that pressure will be released if they return to the owner/trainer. If a horse spooks and shies and even unseats the rider, unless there is continuing danger from flapping tack or other uncertainty, the horse often will come back to the owner/trainer apparently seeking release of the pressure caused by the circumstances.

The study of horse or companion animal psychology is a fascinating ongoing undertaking. We have only begun to understand its mysteries and how horse behavior is woven into coexistence with homo sapiens

Now take a leisurely trip 40 years forward in time and I am a retired veterinarian with time on my hands to ride my horses whenever I so choose. I think my Tennessee Walkers sincerely enjoy getting out to explore and investigate the trails around our mountains and valleys and they usually walk up to me presenting their heads to be haltered. On some occasions I open the tailgate to the horse trailer and the gate to the barn stall and throw the end of the halter rope up over the horse's back. They self-load from their pen into the horse trailer. I close the horse trailer tailgate, start the truck, and we drive off for a horseback adventure. Sometimes on cool or windy days the horses perhaps come galloping in from the back pasture but aren't quite ready to be caught. I can just stand in one place looking the lead horse in the eye and they do one or two or three laps around me snorting and tossing their heads. Then they stop, turn, walk towards me, and lower their heads to be haltered. In my old age I have finally learned enough about communicating with my herd of two horses that we can have relationship that hopefully brings pleasure to all three of us (four counting my dog Piper).

THE GOOD, THE BAD, AND THE UGLY

THE GOOD
This is a funny happy story.

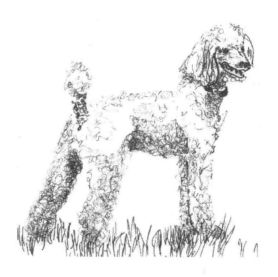

The French poodle actually originated in Germany. It appears in the artwork of Albrecht Durer as early as the 15th century and Francisco Goya in the 18th century. In its full 50 lb. standard size with an ungroomed water-resistant dreadlock hair coat, it was supposedly used to hunt waterfowl. Thus, you would have expected that our standard poodle Elizabeth would have known how to swim and would like the water but this was not to be the case. Too many generations of being walked on a patent leather leash sporting ridiculous haircut must have bred those hunting instincts out. When Liz was young, I took her out to the irrigation canal to encourage her to swim since it is a basic survival instinct that all animals have. I carried her out until I stood shivering waist deep in the water and slowly lowered her down. She tried to climb on top of my head but her feet eventually did begin paddling.

I smiled and said to myself, "That didn't seem to be too difficult."

Then I realized that her body was so long that her hind feet were firmly planted on the canal bottom and only her front feet were paddling. Was she smiling at me?

One thing that got Elizabeth's full attention was the sound and sight of a fish jumping and the ratcheting whine of line being stripped from a fishing reel. When we brought a fish to the bank or into the boat, we had to be careful that Elizabeth didn't try to retrieve it and get caught on the hook herself.

When she was young, we were fishing in a high mountain lake. We had ridden in on our horses with our lunches in the saddlebags. She barked excitedly when she saw our fishing rods and was beside herself when she saw a fish jumping on the end of our line. She finally ran out on a log and launched herself into the cold clear water. We stood there holding our breath and saw her head go under but she came up sputtering doing the dog paddle. I guess she didn't know how to do the breaststroke. Labrador Retrievers know how to stretch out and relax in the water and paddle along strongly and efficiently. Elizabeth, however, looked like a lady desperately trying to keep her fancy hairdo from getting wet. Additionally, she was making no progress towards the shore. I waded out into the lake to rescue my water dog. I was shoulder deep in the water and when I got within reach, she tried to climb up on my shoulders. I supported her belly a little bit and pointed her towards the shore. With this assistance she gradually progressed until she could stagger out to shake off and shower my wife with cold water. We laughed *In Spite of Ourselves*.

On another occasion we were fishing from our boat out in a massive desert irrigation reservoir. By early September the water could warm up and actually reach a pleasant temperature. My wife hooked a nice trout which started jumping wildly on the end of her line. Elizabeth was in the bow of the boat watching intently, dancing, and barking enthusiastically. When the fish got closer to the boat and started jumping again, she couldn't contain herself and launched into the water. When she surfaced you could almost see the look of shock on her face when she discovered she couldn't walk on the water. Her enthusiasm won and she started swimming awkwardly towards the jumping fish hoping she could catch it. We netted the fish and then helped Elizabeth clamber up on the swim tabs on the stern of the boat. She immediately scrambled dripping aboard and pounced on the fish still thrashing on the bottom of the boat. She never really did learn to like the water but she discovered that she could swim across rivers or other water obstacles when the need arose.

Her lifetime goal of becoming a fish catching fish retrieving dog finally came to fruition. We were, as we often did, riding a trail high up in mountain valley. There was a quiet little stream which often dried up to a trickle but there were some quiet pools still full of water. As Elizabeth followed the trail and splashed across a shallow ford, her eye caught the ripple of a small trout trying to escape. She instinctively pounced and perhaps sensing something under her feet plunged her face up into the water and came up with a trout in her teeth caught by the tail. She waded ashore and dropped the fish to get a better purchase only to have it thrash and plop back into the water. If ever there was the look of total bewilderment on a dog's face, that was the moment. We got off our horses to console her. We hugged her, massaged her back, and told her what a good dog she was. We had brought along some weenies to roast over a small fire later in the ride. We tore open the corner of the package and got one out for her. She didn't let it escape. I think that helped ease her disappointment.

In her later years Liz developed a cardiac condition known as atrial fibrillation or Afib. The heart has a rapid irregular rhythm and thus poor blood circulation. The most common result is whole body and system fatigue and shortness of breath. It is often not a major problem but can be debilitating and may be aggravated by the stress of heavy exercise. It first came to our attention on a ride when she started lagging back and was unable to keep up with the horses. When I put my hand and then my ear to her chest the vibration and sound of her arrhythmic heart was alarming. We aborted our ride and I tried carrying her in my arms and then around my neck but it was exhausting and I feared for my own heart. Finally, I remounted my horse and my wife lifted Liz up into my coat padded lap and we headed back to the trail head. About a half hour later she became restless and wanted down. I monitored her heart and she had returned to normal sinus rhythm. I gladly obliged and eased her back down to the ground.

Traveling very slowly we walked with her back to the truck and trailer. We sadly decided that that had to be her last trail ride but we compensated by taking her with us in the truck whenever conditions permitted.

She was able to partially continue her fishing advocation however. We had a small pond in a front flowerbed stocked with Shubunkin fish. Liz could sit by the water and watch the fish swimming below sometimes even sticking her nose in if they got too close.

Now that she is gone to another place, I wonder if rather than chasing butterflies, she has her own aquarium where she can endlessly watch angel fish or other cichlids drift by.

THE BAD

This is not a happy story.

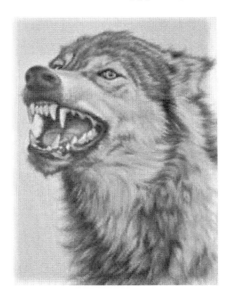

I had been called out to attend a goat with apparent bite wounds on its back and hind legs. I had the address and knew the general vicinity but this was long before the GPS era and the land line telephone directions were rather sketchy; (past the old wooden shed with the donkey hanging around inside, turn left a ways down the road, watch for a shaggy pony standing underneath an oak tree, and then look for the white truck with a flat tire parked by the gray house.) You get the picture! I made a mental note to remind my receptionist that moving objects and unmeasurable distances were not particularly reliable landmarks. I drove anxiously around some quiet lanes and finally saw a woman out working in her garden. She had gardening gloves, bib overalls, rubber boots, and her hair was covered with a kerchief. There was no traffic so I stopped in the middle of the country road and rolled the window.

I shouted out, "Excuse me. Do you know where 827 Oak Lane is"? The lady barely lifted her head and looked at me. About then her raspberry patch exploded and a huge black hairy beast charged my car. I quickly rolled up the window but the dog literally attacked my car. It leaped the roadside ditch and in no time the driver's side window was covered with snot and slobber and I could hear dirty feet and claws stripping the paint off the door. I was afraid I would run over the dog if I drove away so I sat there until the dog finally stopped and retreated to sit alongside his mistress' feet. I collected myself and not being sure if she heard me the first time rolled down the window again and shouted out, "Can you please direct me to 827 Oak Lane?" She just glared at me again with a very hostile frown on her face. I guess I am a slow learner because I got a repeat performance from the dog. By now I'm getting a little hot under the collar and I rolled the window down part way down to tell her to call off her dog so I could drive away and you guessed it, here came the dog for the third time. However, this time I was ready and instinctively without a moment's hesitation or regret, when the dog launched itself in the air at my car, I shoved the car door open. There was a satisfying resounding thwack when the dog collided with my door and was knocked to the ground momentarily stunned. As soon as it recovered it charged again only to be greeted again by my door flying open in his face. This time it retreated growling to his mistress' side. She, understandably, became slightly unglued and unhinged. I suspect she was already unstable and unbalanced. Her kerchief fell off, one of her bib overall shoulder straps came unbuckled, and with her wild hair flying, she charged my car. She was so mad I think she added some spittle to what the dog that already deposited.

After she cooled down a little bit, I cracked open the window only to have her scream at me, "I'm going to call the cops."

I replied, "Please do. I will sit right here exactly on this spot and not move an inch. I will gladly wait for them to arrive. What do you think they will say and do when they get here? I'm sitting here in public right-of-way and your dog left his property to attack me in my car."

I think I saw her shoulders slump a little. She used the sleeve of her sweatshirt to dry off her nose and mouth and stomped away back to her garden. I waited five minutes to give her the opportunity to go to her telephone. She never did. When I finally started my engine to drive away, I saw her stoop down and grab a large clod of dirt and throw it at my car as hard as she could. To this day I do not know what her problem was and why she reacted the way she did. Was she an escapee from an institution? Had she just lost her favorite apple pie recipe? Was it just bad karma? I drove on down the road and began to recognize mailbox numbers and shortly arrived at the goat farm.

The goat owner looked at my car window and door in amazement and asked, "What happened"?

After I gave him a brief explanation, he said, "I know exactly which dog it was and who the crazy owner is."

He had to admit he had been sorely tempted to accidentally swerve and hit it himself. " Fortunately, I'm usually able to control my emotions. I could never live with myself if I did something like that."

He got me a bucket of soapy water and a garden hose and we cleaned up my car but there were deep permanent scratches in the paint that would probably accompany it all the way to the its eventual demise in a junkyard.

Was I happy with myself or proud of my emotional reaction? Certainly not! But I wondered how many schoolchildren, pedestrians, bicyclists, cars, trucks, semi-trucks, airplanes, military convoys, and even freight trains had been attacked by this dog.

The goat recovered nicely from the wounds that might have been inflicted by a very large black hairy dog.

THE UGLY

This is not an ugly story

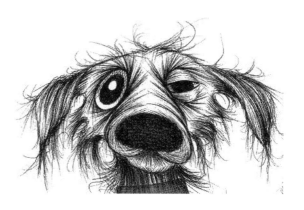

Bugsy was so ugly he was almost adorable. He had eye issues, dental problems, heart defects, respiratory difficulties, jaw abnormalities, leg deformities, joint complications. and even tail irregularities. Otherwise he was in pretty good shape for a Shih Tzu, also known as the Chrysanthemum Dog. However, I don't know of any dog who was more loved and cared for by his owner. Georgina was his guardian wingless angel.

I think it's appropriate to add that Shih Tzus are happy, easy going, and sweet natured little dogs of Tibetan origin They aren't too yappy or demanding and are lively but don't require too much exercise. They love to cuddle on laps or soft pillows and blankets and are definitely creatures of comfort.

Almost all of Bugsy's problems resulted from a genetic disorder called osteochondrodysplasia. At some time in the unknown history of human domestication of the canine species, a mutation apparently appeared involving a defect in bone maturation. The selective breeding to perpetrate these abnormalities resulted in dachshunds, bassets, beagles, and other short-legged breeds.

Imagine a stereotype dog bone with a long shaft and a knobby joint assembly on each end. The knobs migrate away from each end of the shaft leaving a trail of cartilage. Eventually this cartilage turns to bone and this is how bones mature and lengthen. These areas of bone development are called growth plates.

There are parts of the body where pairs of bones mature and develop together: the upper and lower jaw bones, the forelimb radius and ulna, and the hind-limb tibia and fibula. If these pairs of bones don't grow and develop in a coordinated fashion, skeletal abnormalities are the result.

Bugsy had a pug nose because his upper jaw, the maxilla, stopped growing and the lower jaw, the mandible, continued to a relatively normal length. Thus, his lower jaw jutted out and tongue and lower front teeth were not even covered by his upper lip. His upper jaw was so short there was not enough room for all the teeth and they had to rotate sideways to fit in. Hypothetically, the lower jaw could have been shortened. This is sometimes done with the human mandible but would have been extreme in Bugsy's case. We did however have to extract six of his upper premolars. He had a difficult time grasping things between his teeth but learn to use his lower jaw like a scoop when it was time to eat. Even his back teeth were misaligned and he really couldn't chew his food. We teased Georgina and said that she had to chew his food for him.

Additionally, Bugsy's facial and orbital bones we're not normal resulting in a shallower eye socket. Thus, he had the small dog frog eyed appearance. This left his eyes more exposed, and certainly more subject to possible injury and irritation. There is a small glandular structure near the tear duct in the middle corner of the eye called the hardarian gland. If it gets inflamed and enlarged it is called a cherry eye and it can be surgically tucked back into place or even removed if they have adequate additional tearful. Bugsy had more than adequate tear flow so we simply trimmed away this enlarged portion of the gland.

Lastly, he had entropian where the lower eyelid inverts so the eyelashes and the hair on the outside of the lid rub against the cornea. A little *nip and tuck* and both eyes were as good as new. So much for the head redesign and do over.

His front legs were an absolute mess. The radius and ulna are attached to each other and if one grows while the other doesn't, the result is a bowed leg. He was so duck footed he walked like a sea lion and in fact had difficulty even placing his pads on the ground and sometimes even walked on his knuckles. More surgery involved removing a wedge of bone from the longer ulna thus making the radius and ulna the same length and the leg straighter. During the same surgery the paw or carpus was rotated around until the toes pointed forward instead off to each side.

The hind legs were deformed as well with one being considerably worse than the other. We did an angular rotation of his right hind leg get it pointing forward. Prior to that we jokingly said that Bugsy tended to walk in counterclockwise circles because his right leg was able to push harder than the left.

Prior to the leg surgeries, we said, "A predator could never track Bugsy because they couldn't tell if he was coming or going."

Bugsy also had a crazy tail. If the right side of a tail vertebrae grows but the left doesn't then the tail will have a kink in it to the left. Thus, Bugsy had factory-installed permanent tail signals for a left-hand turn. We teased that this was to compensate for his hypothetical tendency to walk in a counter-clockwise direction.

Cats often have kinked tails and people assume that the tail was broken but they have the same hemi-vertebrae condition as Bugsy

Topping off his list of the anomalies, Bugsy had a congenital mitral valve insufficiency. This meant that when his heart contracted the valves were unable to completely close and some of the blood could flow in a reverse direction back towards the lung. The increased blood pressure in the lung caused some fluid leakage into the airways with a resulting persistent lifetime cough. Modern heart medications and diuretics enabled him to lead a fairly active life. The diuretics however necessitated frequent fireplug, telephone pole, and flower garden inspections to relieve himself.

By the time Bugsy was two years old we had resolved most of his problems and he got to enjoy life and we got to enjoy him. Georgina always had him carefully groomed with a little boy blue bow in his top knot and his toenails painted red. I suspect he would have been embarrassed if they were pink. I can't imagine why he was happy to see us but nevertheless he came prancing in the front door with a smile on his funny face and barked enthusiastically when I asked him where his ball was.

His leaky heart finally gave out when he was about 13 years old but we could look back happy to have given him 11 years or

77 dog years of painless active life. We had Georgina bring in Bugsy's successor Pricilla for a pre-purchase health examination to make sure she had all the appropriate parts in all the right places.

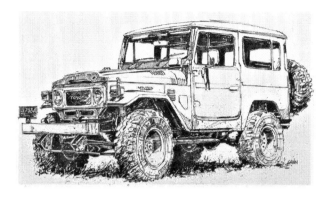

THE CAMPING TRIP

It had been a busy 12 months. I had finished my final semester of Vet School, my National Veterinary Board Examinations, and graduated from the Washington State University College of Veterinary Medicine. I was now a real live Doctor of Veterinary Medicine and had even learned how to spell *vet er i nar i an*. I had taken the provincial veterinary medical board exams required to practice veterinary medicine in British Columbia, Canada and applied for and received landed immigrant status. There was a shortage of veterinarians in Canada so the whole process took an amazingly short six weeks to complete. Canada welcomed applicants with skills when a shortage existed.

I started as an associate in late August and 2 months later I had been invited to become a partner. At 6 months my partner traveled back to his German homeland to visit his ailing father and I was left to run the practice solo for six weeks. I spend a lot of evening hours in my veterinary reference books confirming how to do procedures I had never done before.

That fall we got pregnant. I never did figure out how that happened. In June we became the proud parents of Jeffery. He was overdue so our family doctor Mike, after consulting with an obstetrician, decided to induce labor. We waited all day and all evening but Jeffrey must have been a little shy and still didn't want to make an appearance so I was finally sent home to bed. At 2 in the morning the phone rang and I hurried down to the delivery room. It was similar to my getting up in the middle of the night for a veterinary emergency only this time it was my family. I walked through the hospital door at 2:15am, by 2:20am I had my mask, gown, and gloves on, and by 2:40am there was another person in the room. I'm not sure where he came from.

In the months prior to this, for obvious reasons, we had been staying pretty close to home but Linda recovered quickly from her pregnancy and when Jeff was 6 weeks old, we decided we were ready for a short car camping trip. My practice had a work schedule where we worked 10 days and then were off for a four-day weekend. This was perfect for the camping and outdoor activities we enjoyed and the four days were almost like a mini-vacation.

Not far away was Harrison Lake with a fairly famous resort called Harrison Hot Springs. We knew they had opened up a new road on the west side of the lake for future logging and decided to go exploring and camping there. We loaded up the tent, sleeping bags, cooking gear and enough food for a few days. We added a six pack of Kokanee beer and a package of Oreo Cookies for good measure. Our 15 lb. Cockapoo Fricha was already warming up the driver's seat. I have to admit it was convenient not to have to bring any formula or means of warming up baby bottles. Linda had all the baby feeding equipment and supplies well under control.

We pulled out on the Lougheed Highway and headed east towards Harrison Hot Springs. We stopped at the resort for a coffee, Coke and a bagel. I was never man enough to drink coffee so my default drink was Coke. In no time we were bouncing down a new logging road in our FJ40 Toyota Land Cruiser. Soon we passed through an area that had been previously harvested and on into virgin old growth timber. Linda cradled baby Jeff in her lap and the jouncing seemed to aid his slumber. This was before the era of mandatory baby seats and we thought we were being good protective parents by securing Jeff in his mother's arms. He, like most other children of that era, managed to survive their parent's safety mistakes and grow to productive adulthood.

We stopped alongside a rushing stream for lunch and built a tiny fire to roast our weenies. When slathered with mustard and relish with some shredded cheese on top, they were pretty tasty. When they built the road, they had put in some temporary log bridges across the major streams. A heavy spring runoff, however, had washed out the bridge. Out of curiosity I waded out into it to discover it was only about knee deep.

"Should we keep going?" I asked.

Linda a was young and adventurous women so she said, "Why not?"

Leaving her and baby Jeff on the bank I cautiously proceeded to drive into the river. It was a little rough but doable so I came back to collect my family and we proceeded on into the wilderness.

The next two fords were pretty easy but the third one looked a little less certain. The temporary bridge was still there but the approaches on either end were pretty eroded. That became a challenge that a *guy* couldn't refuse. Using driftwood, small logs, rocks, and gravel we reconstructed an approach to the bridge and our trusty Toyota was able to scramble up and cross over the bridge. When I drove off the other end of the bridge we stopped and looked back to see that our passing had disrupted more of the bridge footing and it looked like it could collapse. We checked the map found that we were more than halfway through to the remote town of Lillooet.

It was late in the day and the sun just starting to set so we decided to camp there. We built a big fire, set up the tent and grilled hamburger when the fire had burned down. We looked back across the river to see a small band of deer coming down to drink and later a moose with her wobbly calf. They didn't seem surprised or startled by our presence in their forest domain. During the night we were serenaded by coyotes and spotted owls hooting from the trees. There were a few very disturbing crashes and thumps in the night but baby Jeff slept right through it and we just snuggled deeper into our sleeping bags. Those Sasquatches sure could be noisy! We had zipped our two bags together making one giant sleeping bag and put our son between us. I guess the jury is still out on whether mothers should sleep with their babies but we all survived. It certainly made it easier when Jeffrey woke up hungry in the middle of the night.

We woke up to a dew-covered tent which made it a little tricky staying dry when dressing and getting out. There were still some coals in the fire so in no time at all we had the hotcake griddle positioned and ready. In the morning daylight I re-examined the bridge and thought that it might be possible to return but there was certainly some obvious risk. The Sasquatches must have erased their tracks.

The map indicated we weren't too many miles from First Nation communities and we therefore hoped for more established permanent roads. We were at a very critical point of our adventure because the gas tank was reading slightly below half full. There would have been enough to retrace our route back to civilization but not enough if we found ourselves in the middle of a small river after a bridge collapsed. So, we loaded everything up with baby in arms and our dog Fricha helping drive from her position on the middle of the front bench seat. The roads got better and we started passing some houses and small cattle ranches on First Nation reserve land but we were not finding any gas stations.

As the gas gauge continue to drop, we finally passed a sign that said Lillooet 16 kilometers and we finally knew that we were not going to be stranded out of gas in the wilderness. But then we drove around a corner and there in front of us was a manned barricade across the road but all the people were on our side of the barrier. When we drove up behind them, they were certainly startled to see us. They were all First Nation young men and we realized that we had been driving across their reserve.

Canadian First Nation people like Native Americans have had much of their culture and land stripped away. The people were lobbying the government to reclaim more of their land but with limited success. It turns out the main road through the area traveled across their Reserve and to protect their rights they had blocked the road. This prevented the British Columbia government from crossing the reservation to access crown land on the other side. Politically, things were at a loggerhead.

That was the situation we had unwittingly stumbled into. I got out of my vehicle to talk to them and they seemed unfriendly and less than pleased to see me.

They asked me, "Where did you come from? How did you get here?"

I said, "I just drove up from Harrison Hot Springs along the lake shore."

They said, "How did you do that? There is no road through there."

I said, "There is now because they pushed it through last fall and here I am."

"Well, we're only letting Lillooet band members drive through," they said determinedly.

I explained, "I am almost out of gas and I'm just a foolish American out on a camping trip with my wife and baby. You can see she's nursing him back in the Toyota."

They grumbled and arguing amongst themselves for a while leaving me up in the air.

I said, "I've got about $50, a six pack of Kokanee beer, and a package of Oreo Cookies. Would that be an adequate trade to bypass your barricade?"

There was a little more grumbling and arguing and finally a young man who seemed to be leader with a big smile on his face walked up said, "Well! You can keep your money but we'll take your beer and cookies."

We drove on into Lillooet and filled our gas tank. From there it was easy going on nice paved highways through Pemberton, past the world-famous Whistler destination ski resort, and down to the salt water at Squamish. We then drove past the BC ferry landing at Horseshoe Bay, the Lions Gate Bridge, Stanley Park, through Vancouver, and back up the Lougheed Highway to be home again.

The next morning my veterinary partner ask me, "What did you do with your four days off?"

I said, "Oh! We just went for a scenic drive and did a little camping. Nothing too exciting."

When Jeff grew up, we told him the story about how we almost became stranded in the wilderness 30 miles from civilization and were almost captured by a friendly band of North American natives who could have kidnapped him. When he turned 16, we gave him the old Toyota Land Cruiser so he could go out and explore and create his own adventures. The old Cruiser was 7 years older than he was.

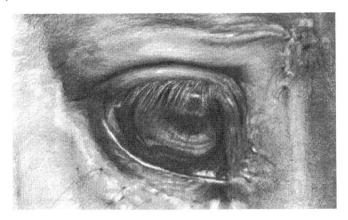

THE EQUINE EYE

The equine eye is a truly amazing organ, especially adapted for a grazing fright and flight type animal. Horses have the largest eyes for their body size of all the mammals. Scientific studies of horse eyes are sometimes accomplished by temporarily attaching light emitting diodes to sedated horse corneas and then measuring the response of the retina and optic nerve. Intensity (brightness), wavelength (color), motion, and patterns can be altered to determine eye and retina response.

The function and response of the eye greatly influences equine behavior. Because of the large size of the pupil (the opening in the iris) the horse eye can capture six times more light than the human eye and can thus see and navigate in almost total darkness (by starlight?) They have a tapetum lucidum, a mirror like pigment behind the retina, which reflects light (photons) back through the retina thus doubling the light received by the rod receptors in the retina. This is the structure which gives nocturnal animals glowing eyeshine in your headlights. The retina is covered with rods (for black and white) and cones (for color) which are light receptors that translate light into a nerve impulse which the optic nerve sends to the brain. Horses have a greater density of rods in their retina than humans thus further enhancing night vision. Rods are amazingly receptive to light (at levels of one photon) and especially to light motion. This is why you can perceive things in dim light better if you don't look directly at them. You are of tricking your eye and brain to see perceived motion.

If you look into a horse's eye you will see a structure attached to the 6:00 o'clock area of the pupil which looks like the tree logo of public television's Nature program. This is the corpra nigra. In bright sunlight the horse's eye can collect so much light that the horse can be temporarily blinded. The pupil, unlike that of the human eye, can take 15 – 30 minutes to completely dilate or constrict while adjusting to dramatic light intensity changes. In bright light, the corpra nigra quickly enlarges by blood engorgement thus acting like the sun visor on your car windshield and reducing the amount of light reaching the retina. What is the significance of this for us as horse owners? Horses adapt to light intensity changes slowly and may not want to walk into a dark trailer or barn or down trails with deep shadow. Let them take their time (you can't wait 15 minutes obviously) and proceed when they are ready.

You can also have trust in your horse. I have ridden literally all night on moonless overcast nights and had my horse never miss a step. They have even stopped when there was a low hanging branch I couldn't see. Horses, like deer, are blinded by bright car lights so be careful when riding your horse down the middle of I-90 at midnight. Does your arena or barn have a bright sunlit doorway or areas or darkness or places shaded by trees? These factors can affect how your horse works.

As mentioned, the horse eye has a greater density of rods but less cones than the human eye. While the human eye has three types of cones in the retina the horse has only two. They can see blue and green wavelengths but not red. (The bird has four types of cones and can even see ultraviolet wavelengths). Horse color vision has been described to be much like red/green color blindness in humans. Their natural habitat is mainly greens without many red stop signs or flashing emergency lights. What is the significance? If you are into making obstacles for your horse, you might want to color them so they contrast with the natural environment. Red obstacles are poorly perceived while blue and white stripes would really stand out. I am color blind and *hunter red* is a joke for me. However, I rarely shoot hunters dressed in yellow or blue.

A horse's pupil is somewhat rectangular in shape while the human pupil is round. Additionally, there is an increase in rods in the horse's retina corresponding to the pupil shape. Thus, the horse has an area of visual acuity like a car low beam headlight. Depending on the study, horses are said to have 20/30 or even 20/60 vision which means what we see at 60 feet, a horse needs to be at 20 feet to see it clearly. Dogs have 20/50, cats 20/75 and rats 20/300. See who catches who? Rats only see things close up and must rely on smell and hearing to survive while cats with better vision have the advantage.

Horse's eyes are set widely on the side of their head so they can see 350 degrees. There is however, a blind spot over their rump and in front of their nose for about 3 to 4 feet. Their peripheral vision is relatively poor and they can't rotate their eyes in their sockets as well as humans. The human brain can take our binocular vision and merge it into one picture. The horse only has about 65 degrees of binocular vision directly in front while the rest is monocular lateral vision which their brain doesn't merge into one picture. Can you imagine watching a different TV channel with each eye? A horse could.

The horse's ability to accommodate or focus is also limited. Like us, if we wore bi/tri/quadra focal eyeglasses, they need to move their head and thus their cone of vision to maximize the clarity of what they are looking at. What is the significance?

1. Horses have high visual sensitivity to motion but poor acuity. Thus, they are startled by motion and must turn their head to see the source of the motion. Windy days might be a nightmare because all the moving grass and bushes might hide a predator such as the Big Bad Wolf, a sasquatch, or Smokey The Bear. They are herd animals, so if the horse in front on a trail ride startles so might the rest of the followers.

2. They are blind for 10 degrees over their rump so approach a horse from the side and announce your approach vocally. Your horse may not be comfortable as *tail gunner* or **drag** on a trail ride. He may be timid, but also knows he is vulnerable to attack from the blind spot behind. Do you back your horse out of the trailer? He is blind as he steps backward searching for that last step down.

3. They can't see directly in front of their nose for 3 to 4 feet and if you lead them from directly in front, they might

accidentally step on you. They use their sense of smell and feel to help navigate this blind spot. Trimming their sensitive muzzle hairs is giving them a slight handicap. Notice how they investigate you with their sense of smell at close range and almost prehensile lips. Notice a horse's whiskers but also the other dense strangely matted hair on their muzzle which is also highly touch sensitive.

4. We like to **collect the head** in arena or show riding because it makes the horse more attractive but are thus limiting how well the horse sees and therefore moves. They need a full range of head motion laterally and vertically to maximize use of their cone of greatest visual acuity as well as to balance their body. The horse points its head at what it wants to see. Notice how stadium jumpers give their horse its head the last few strides before the jump. The horse needs this to see the jump. Calf ropers all seem to use heavy tie downs on their horses to keep the head out of the way of the rope but thus inhibit vision and balance. At least the roping arena has consistently good footing.

5. On the trail, horses drop their head at water crossings or areas of poor footing but lift them to see the deer in the distance. With their head down, they feel vulnerable to predators and with their head up they are more susceptible to stumbling. (Damn bifocals!) Anything that affects vision can, of course, have an effect your horse's behavior. The cornea, aqueous humor, lens and vitreous humor must allow the passage of light. Injury to the cornea often makes it cloudy (edema). Uveitis (inflammation of the vascular tract of the eye) can cause changes to the lens or humors such as cataracts or infiltrates (blood components like RBCs or WBCs) into the humors. Cysts on the iris, retinal degeneration, or injury caused lens movements also all affect vision. The lens is suspended like a trampoline in the eye by the ciliary body. The ciliary body produces the aqueous humor and is also the muscle that changes the lens shape to allow focusing. Head or eye trauma can damage the support structures of the lens and allow it to move out of place (luxate) in the globe.

Some of us have dealt with blind horses. The ability of some horses to adapt to loss of vision is truly amazing. Don't change a blind horse's environment. Put different sounding bells on pasture mates. Supply a **seeing eye goat** pasture buddy if necessary. Keep food and water easily available 24/7 and enjoy them as wonderful, appreciative pasture pets or ornaments. They thrive on attention and grooming. Unfortunately, some are unable to handle the stress and are a danger to themselves and to the people around them.

Humans like variety and novelty in their pets. Horse iris or eye color is usually brown. Blue, hazel, green, and amber also occur and may be selected in breeding choices. There appears to be no increased risk of cancer in these more unusual eye color patterns. Keep in mind that these alternate light eye colors may make the eye more sensitive to light which might manifest itself in increased tear flow and discharge at the corner of the eye. Totally white pigmentation of the sclera (white of the eye) also has the same effect.

Given the option, I would choose a brown eyed girl (I mean horse).

Don't tell my girlfriend!

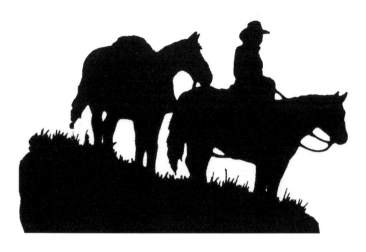

HONEYMOON

"What would you like to do for our honeymoon?" I asked my bride to be.

Her response was instantaneous. "Can we go on a horse pack trip?"

She knew that I had spent many summers living in the woods working for the USFS and wanted me to share the experience with her. The price was right. Free. Reservations? None were required. The accommodations were spacious: the whole out of doors. Gratuities were not an issue because it was self-service. Travel time was minimal because the destination was virtually in our backyard. Travel itself was also extremely easy because we had the unlimited use of the self-driving 1 horsepower model and we only had to sit back and enjoy the scenery.

I said with a smile on my face, "You're certainly making this difficult for me. Well at least that's settled."

I called my good friend Louie. We had spent many hours working together as packers for the forest service.

"Louie. I'm getting married. My wife to be wants to do our honeymoon up in the wilderness. Could I rent your horse Packy?" I asked.

There was a long worrisome pause in the conversation. Then Louie said, "Gosh Fred. I'm sorry but I don't think that I can let you do that." I knew Louie had to have a good reason but I certainly felt deflated nevertheless.

There was another long pause and then Louie said, "However, if you can catch him out in the pasture, he needs the exercise and you are more than welcome to borrow him. Also, my camp up at the lake is vacant and I would be honored to let you use it for the week. On second thought, there will be a small charge: How about a batch of your cowboy cookies. There's lots of firewood and I just took up a fresh propane tank for the cook stove. Have a great time!"

It didn't take too long to switch out of a suit and wedding dress into boots, Levi's, and long sleeve shirts. My head felt better covered by my old felt western hat. At the trailhead we unloaded the horses from the trailer and saddled them. They were as anxious to get going as we were. A weeks' worth of supplies were quickly mantied up and loaded onto Packy's Decker packsaddle.

When Louie waved goodbye from the trailhead he said, "Rats! I forgot to bring the rice and the tin cans to tie onto the horse's tails. That's what you're supposed to do when someone drives away on their honeymoon. Right?"

It was a three-hour ride into the camp and as promised the wall tent, fire wood and pit, Coleman lantern, and propane cook stove were waiting for us. A Douglas squirrel scolded us from the spruce tree and a mouse scurried back into the shelter of the tent. After securing and giving the horses grain, we worked together in our outdoor kitchen to grill a chuck steak, fry some potatoes in the cast iron pan, and toss a fresh green salad. A celebratory glass of local red wine and Oreo cookies put the final touch on our first meal together as a married couple.

The next day we went fishing in the nearby lake and its outlet river. We caught and carefully released some nice rainbow trout but decided to call it a day when black threatening clouds began building in the nearby mountain peaks. We got back to camp just in time and were thankful to enjoy the shelter of the wall tent when the rain began coming down. The sound on the tent roof was mesmerizing and called for a nap. Later we cooked inside with the light of the Coleman lantern and played a few hands of hearts before deciding to crawl into the warmth of our sleeping bags.

Toward midnight the storm changed intensity with a heavy downpour and serious thunder and lightning. If you count the seconds between the flash and crash and divide that by 5 you got the number of miles to the lightning strike. At first it was 15 seconds or three miles. Then it was 10 seconds or 2 miles. Then it was 5 Seconds.

When it got to 2 seconds and less my wife, trying to remain calm, said, "Wow! That sounds pretty close."

Eventually the flash and crash were virtually simultaneous and we knew the storm was right in our front yard. We had tied the horses under the rain deflecting branches of a giant spruce tree and I cautiously picked out beneath the tent flaps to make sure that our three horses weren't glowing in the dark. They stood there trembling but had not yet been turned into barbecue. The storm gradually drifted off but then the water started trickling into our tent.

My wife said, "You're the camp engineer. I think we have a plumbing problem," so I grabbed a Pulaski and quickly excavated a trench to deflect the flood waters away.

As the woods gradually hushed, we drifted off to sleep listening do the quiet thumping sounds of the horse's hooves as our self-driving vehicles shifted around and settled in for the night. We awoke in the morning to bright sunlight and bird songs. Even though the sun was out and drying things off, we essentially spent the morning in gentle rain showers because the grass, bushes and, and trees all sprinkled on you when you got too near.

After a breakfast of oatmeal, bacon, eggs, and Dutch oven biscuits, we saddled up to explorer our little piece of heaven. Packy felt pretty sassy because he got to travel along unhindered by a rider or pack.

We followed a trail into a side valley. After some steep switchbacks we passed a cascading waterfall and then the trail leveled out and opened up into a round glacier carved valley filled with grassy meadows, vine maple thickets, giant spruce trees, and Alpine and Silver fir. It had been a fairly severe winter with heavy snowfall. Even though it was mid-July, there were still patches of snow and drifts in the shade of the trees. A sunny side trail switch backed up a southern exposed hillside. We tied our horses at the top and proceeded on foot across a snow field towards a lake hidden in a glacial cirque. The snow was firm so we could walk fairly comfortably on top but had to squint because the bright sunlight was reflected off the snow.

I paused to catch my breath and looked back to discover that my wife had disappeared. "Where did she go?" I wondered. I quickly retraced my steps and looked down into a hole. She was in the bottom standing in a shallow stream with an embarrassed expression on her face. The steam had melted out the bottom of a snowbank and she had been unlucky enough to cross a snow bridge in an area that would not support her weight. After determining that she was not hurt I threw a snowball down at her. She tried to smile but was obviously not pleased with my twisted sense of humor.

After extracting her from her dilemma, we continued on the frozen over snow covered lake. There was a swimming pool sized area of open water that must have been fed by warm spring water.

I had brought along a lightweight trout fishing pole for my wife and she playfully said, "Don't you know how to put that thing together?"

I pretended to hurry and put it in her hands. Every time she cast a lure into this water the fish virtually fought over which one would be the first to get hooked. I suspect that the winners of these contests regretted their eagerness. Unfortunately, they were not the only animals that were hungry after a winter of no food. Mrs. Mosquito and her countless cousins were also in attendance.

It turns out mosquitoes breed for the last time in the fall and all the males, having been lucky or not, die. However, these female mosquitoes have accumulated glycerol, an antifreeze like product, in their system that prevents them from being destroyed by ice crystals that might forum in their bodies. When temperature rises only a few degrees above freezing in the spring, they warm up and hover around like blood thirsty vampire drones. Blood has the protein necessary for them to produce eggs.

Swatting and slapping, we were driven from our blindingly bright crystalline retreat back down to the comfort of our valley camp. There is something unique about my blood type and body smell that the mosquitoes don't like so I'm not horribly hounded by them. However, my wife was not so lucky. I asked her if I needed to call the American Red Cross and see if they had blood of her type for a transfusion. In spite of liberal applications of DEET and wearing light-colored clothing my wife wins the mosquito lottery every time.

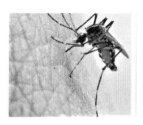

Having had a strenuous workout the day before we decided that we and the horses deserved a day of rest in the camp. After a delightful breakfast of hot cakes augmented by some early tangy thimble berries, we mixed a batch of bread and set it out to rise in a patch of warm morning sunshine. Realizing that the horses needed more than just grain, we jumped on them bareback and rode off to a nearby meadow to let them forage. We decided it was better to let them graze while we held the end of their halter ropes rather than risk the chance of them returning 11 miles back down to the trailhead on auto pilot. It was relaxing to sit on a log reading and listening to them munch as they delicately plucked out choice blades of grass from among the other inedible plants. The dog prowled around the meadow perimeter trying to sneak up on unsuspecting chipmunks. I think the chipmunks won the staring contest. After a couple of hours, the horses stopped grazing indicated that their gas tanks were full, so we jumped back on for the short ride back to the camp. The woods were quiet, the sun was warm, the birds were napping, the bees were humming, and it was a perfect time for a short snooze in the quiet of the tent. When we awoke the bread had risen and we buried the Dutch oven in the warm ashes left from the fire. 60 minutes later, trying not to drool, we lifted the lid to inspect our handiwork. It was perfectly round, golden brown, and irresistible. Half an hour later, a half cube of butter and the whole loaf of fresh baked bread turned up missing. I wonder what happened to them?

The rest of the week passed all too quickly. A mule deer doe brought her spotted fawn in to investigate our camp every evening. I hope they enjoyed the spilled grain left by the horses. We caught a few more fish, laughed at the foolish antics of a ruffled grouse hen as she clucked and guided her brood of chicks under the nearby pine trees. We fed Camp Robbers hotcake remnants when they flew down from nearby branches to steal them from our outstretched hands.

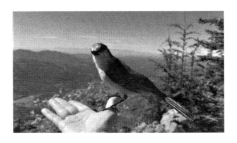

On the last day the dog and horses seem to anticipate the return to civilization and they were eager to go. Their two-legged companions did not share their enthusiasm. We restocked the wood pile, swept out the tent, and used a fallen spruce branch to rake the campsite. We wanted to leave it in better condition than we found it.

The eager horses quickly carried us downriver to the trailhead where are we had to sadly accept reality that our horse pack trip honeymoon and come to an end.

Packy was returned to his pasture and position of mountain pack horse emeritus. All too soon Monday morning arrived and my veterinary office staff had a full slate of farm calls, surgeries, and office visits. Later that week when we were putting equipment away and doing laundry you could still smell the rich heavy aroma of wood smoke on our clothes and I observed three large wood ants drop out on the garage floor when I shook out the sleeping bags.

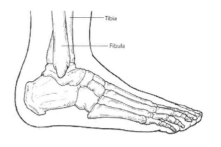

PRACTICING MEDICINE WITHOUT A LICENSE #1

"I'm so frustrated and mad I could cry. We hiked all the way in here two days ago on Monday and found a perfect campsite up near the lake. There was a beautiful breeze off the water that kept the mosquitoes away. We caught enough fish for dinner and a doe with her spotted fawn came right into camp looking for a handout. I was puttering around camp yesterday and stumbled on a slippery rock and found myself sitting on my ankle. I hoped it was just a sprain but I spent a really miserable night. When I got up this morning my ankle was swollen and black and blue and I couldn't even pull my boot on. We remembered passing your camp on the way in so I sent my husband down to see if you were home."

That was how I met Bob and Barbara. I later found out they were in their mid-50s but they looked like mid-30s. They had backpacking down to a fine art and I know they left all their campsites cleaner and in a more natural state than they found them.

Bob had luckily found me at my camp as I was starting to pack up for my return to civilization for my two days off. I had gotten up early to feed the horses, split some fire wood, and tidy up the camp. I had spent a few minutes watching the chicken-like antics of a mama grouse and her 3 chicks scratching in the dirt for grain near the horse's feed box. When Bob found me and explained their predicament, I put my tools away and we hurried back up to their camp by the lake to try and figure out what to do.

Barbara somehow managed a wistful smile when she said "Welcome to Bob and Barbara's B&B. If you're hungry there are some leftover hot cakes there by the fire. I was going to feed them to the camp robbers."

Barb's ankle was indeed ugly. It was so swollen you could also almost imagine it throbbing with every beat of her heart. We sat around the smoldering remnants of their morning fire for a confab. One could only hope that the sound of small waves lapping at the pebbles on the lakeshore would reduce the anxiety level.

At that point in time the Alpine Lakes Wilderness Area was not finalized and it was still legal to fly in and land a float plane.

I suggested, "I wonder if we could fly Barb out?" However, there on the valley floor my government radio was useless and would still be 30 years before satellite cell phones appeared.

"Have you ever ridden a horse?" I asked.

Barb replied, "No I never have. I think I'm afraid of them."

"Well I guess we need to find out. It seems like horseback is the best way to get you out of here," I said.

But we needed some way to stabilize her ankle. We looked at camping equipment, padded sticks, and anything at hand but nothing seemed to fit the bill to make a splint. Bob was repacking their camping equipment and was in the process of deflating the air mattresses. It occurred to me that one of them might do the job. We wrapped her foot, ankle, and lower leg in the air mattress and when we puffed and puffed until we were red in the face it provided a surprisingly comfortable and rigid support for her injured extremity. We wrapped some parachute cord around it to finish our handicraft. It looked pretty silly but no one was laughing.

I hurried back down the trail and closed up my camp. Part of my job as Wilderness Ranger was to collect and pack out trash and cans from along the trails and from the campsites. Thus, my pack animals often carried full loads out of the woods as well as in. The plan was to put Barb on my saddle horse and the pack horses would carry the trash and her pack. That left Bob on foot carrying his pack and leading the pack horses and me in front on foot leading Barb who would be riding on my horse.

When I got back to the lake camp with my saddle horse, Barbara was sitting on a log waiting. There was a worried smile on her face.

She said, "I'm not sure what worries me the most. Riding a horse or sitting here with what might be a broken ankle."

Trying to use my most comforting reassuring tone of voice I said, "It'll be just fine, Barb. There's nothing to worry about at all."

After a few false starts we finally got Barb seated in the saddle of my horse. We were feeding him some of the leftover hot cakes to keep him occupied during this process.

She looked like she was on the verge of tears but as she sat there a grin of accomplishment slowly spread across her face. I led my saddle horse around a little bit by his halter while she sat on board while strangling the saddle horn with both hands.

Eventually we returned to my camp where I finished loading the pack horses and down the trail we went. It took us about four hours walking slowly to get back to the trailhead. When Barb needed a rest Bob and I lifted her out of the saddle where she could lie down on the ground on our spread-out coats. We were very appreciative of the fact that she was only a 130 lb. package.

When we got to the trailhead and their car, I got a quick hug from Barb and a firm handshake from Bob and they waved goodbye as they disappeared down the road towards their home in the Seattle area. About two weeks later a postcard showed up at the Rangers office in Cle Elum addressed to the Waptus Lake Wilderness Ranger.

It said, "Thank you and your horse for the rescue. Barbara indeed has a broken ankle but since there was no displacement, she will only need to wear a fiberglass foot cast for 3 months. We hope she will heal in time for one or two more hikes before snowfall and the end of the camping season. See you next summer?" Signed, B & B

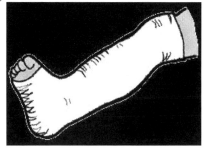

$$$$$

He must have been waiting. We'd only had the lights turned on for 5 minutes when he came through the front door. Rumpled blond hair with a cowlick, a few freckles on his nose, a t-shirt ready for a cycle through the washing machine, and sneakers with one frayed shoelace trailing on the floor.

The boy said, "I brought my kitty in to get it fixed."

Cindy my receptionist said, "Did you have an appointment?"

"No! Did I need one?" was the answer.

"Well that's usually customary but perhaps we can fit you in. Is your mother here?"

"No!"

"What is your name?"

"My name is Robert but I prefer Bobby. I'm eleven and a half years old. I'll be twelve on November 9th."

"How did you get here?"

"I brought my kitty down on my bicycle," was the quick answer.

"Is this okay with your mother, Bobby? How are you going to pay for it?"

Bobby anxiously blurted out, "My mother said last week I could have a kitten if I saved up enough money to get it fixed. I've been mowing all the lawns in the neighborhood. Yesterday this lady was giving kittens away in the Safeway parking lot and she said I could have one. I've saved up $13 already. Mommy hasn't seen it yet."

That's when Cindy came to find me hoping I would rescue her from her financial and emotional dilemma.

I was trapped. It was two against one and I was a pretty easy mark.

I told Cindy, "I guess we can always fit another kitten surgery in. I sure hope it's a little tom."

Bobby asked, "How much will it cost?"

"Do you know if it's a little boy or a little girl, Bobby?" said Cindy.

"No! But I think it's a little boy because he has two little round things back there."

59

After I gave in to Cindy's silent plea for help, we discussed the matter and agreed that people take better care of things if they pay something for them. We decided the cost of a neuter and vaccination would be $10 leaving him with $3 change to get some kitten food.

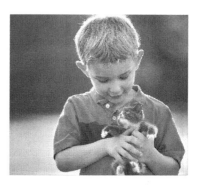

That afternoon a woman came in with Bobby to pick up the kitten. She had tears in her eyes when she said, "Thank you so much for helping me and Bobby. I'm a single mother working two jobs and things are pretty tight. Bobby is such a helpful and good little boy I just couldn't bear the thought of having to tell him NO. He's becoming my man around the house."

I said, "Bobby's sincere effort and honesty and your thanks are all the payment that is required."

That reminded me of an old saying from a long gone cowboy friend of mine. He liked to say, "Thanks a million, until you're better paid."

Recalling this story from many years back brings to mind another medical dilemma that has always troubled me. There are four parts to this problem.

1. The cost of a medical education is high and many students graduate with significant student loan debt. They need an adequate income to pay off this debt.

2. Medical technology has dramatically improved over the years but the cost has also risen proportionally.

3. There are numerous older affordable medical techniques that worked more than adequately in the past but they have been supplanted by more technical and more expensive modern techniques.

4. If a doctor used an older technique and the outcome was not as expected he could be guilty of failure to meet contemporary practice standards.

In a perfect world a client could be given the option of using an older more affordable approach to a medical problem. In veterinary medicine often the best approaches for a medical issue exceed the ability of a client to pay. Older practitioners often have alternate approaches that a client can afford but they are used at the risk of not meeting practice standards should the approach fail. It's interesting to note that these older successful and affordable techniques are no longer even taught as part of the veterinary medical curriculum.

Here is another antidote from my past as a veterinary medical practitioner.

Hank was an athletic muscular Labrador Pitbull mix. He had all the good qualities of the Labrador Retriever and none of the undesirable qualities of a Pitbull but his enthusiastic approach to life left hm prone to leap before he looked. He crossed into traffic one day without looking and was struck by the bumper of a Honda Civic. The Honda won. He made it into the clinic on three legs but still had a grin on his face. An x-ray documented a mid-shaft fracture to his humerus; the bone between his shoulder and elbow. There are a multitude of surgical approaches to repair this fracture but most are technical, complicated, and thus prove to be quite expensive. The apparatus must hold the bones in the proper configuration and prevent rotation.

Surgical intervention with steel rods, plates, and connecting devices are fairly recent inventions. Such approaches were not technically feasible in the past and yet veterinarians were able to devise means of setting bones in such a way that they could heal.

The best approaches were well beyond the financial means of Hank's owner's young growing family. They were shocked when I told them the best modern approach would cost at least $1,000. I also had to inform them that I was not an orthopedic surgery specialist and my first recommendation had to be to offer them very best that was available for Hank. It would have been a referral to a specialist who would have to charge at least $2,000.

"Both those fees are out of reach for us. Isn't there something we could at least try and that we could afford?" asked Hank's owners.

Some bones such as the scapula, the ribs, and the humerus are so surrounded by a circle of muscle tissue that, should they become broken, surgery is often not necessary. All that needs to be done is to stabilize the bones in the relatively normal position.

With Hank's owners' consent, we proceeded. We taped his upper arm back against his rib cage making a tape body cast that incorporated the broken bones. Then bending padded flat bars of aluminum strap into a J shape which we hung upside down over his back, we were able to support the elbow and lower leg in such a way that it could not reach the ground or support any weight. Six rolls of 2-inch-wide white adhesive tape, a little bit of black magic marker ink to draw a large smiley face and Hank was good to go.

The good news to Hank's family was the $300 price tag. The result 8 weeks later, was perhaps not as perfect as it might have been with surgical intervention but six months later you could not tell he had ever been injured.

I didn't get rich during this interaction with Hank and his family but in the long run, I had the immense satisfaction of knowing we'd come up with a way to make fixing Hank an affordable proposition for his family.

The medical and financial needs of the doctor, the patient, the medicine and equipment providers, and the patient's family too often are coming into conflict. Sometimes the problem is irreconcilable. Most frequent cause of personal bankruptcy is a medical emergency. Sometimes the only solution is a compromise on the part of all parties concerned. The world is certainly a happier friendlier place when this is accomplished with a smile of generosity and compassion on everyone's face.

A farmer can fix anything with some baling wire. A mechanic only needs a large adjustable wrench. A cowboy can make do with rawhide. I can do pretty well with a large quantity of white medical adhesive tape.

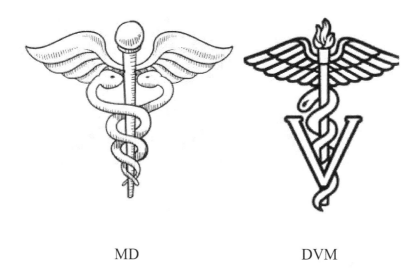

MD   DVM

PRACTICING MEDICINE WITHOUT A LICENSE #2

I never did learn his name. Since we were the only people there, names did not seem to be necessary under the circumstances. He was just a nice guy about 45 years old who came into my camp one evening asking for my help.

While studying and training to become a veterinarian, I spent my summers working as a Wilderness Ranger for the USFS. My summer home was 11 miles up a mountain river valley near a place called Waptus Lake. My job entailed campsite construction and maintenance, light trail work, and just being a government presence in the Alpine Lakes area.

I had spent the day with my saddle horse and pack animals up a nearby side valley at a lake where I cleaned and improved the campsites and cut logs out of the trail. I mantied up the collected cans and trash and tired, hungry, and dirty, I arrived back at my camp about 6 p.m. I had just started my dinner cooking on my outside fire and washed my face in icy cold creek water when my surprise visitor arrived.

He tried to smile when he said, "Hello," but you could see his heart was not really in it. I reached out with my right hand to shake hands when I realized that his right hand was tucked into a sling made from modifying his t-shirt.

He lowered himself into my camp chair with a sigh and I said, "Looks like you have a problem."

He explained that he had probably hiked too long and too far and arrived exhausted at his prospective campsite. As he was taking his pack off, he tripped and stumbled and fell on his shoulder.

"I don't know what I did but it sure hurts," he said. "I came past your empty camp earlier and hoped that you might return in the evening so here I am."

I sat and talked with him for a while until he stopped sweating and some color returned to his face. We got the improvised sling off and his arm hung painfully and uselessly at his side. He tried not to scream while I gently poked and prodded to see what I could learn. When you compared the two shoulders it was obvious that is right arm was rotated forward towards his chest. Using my Superman X-ray vision, I determined that there weren't any broken bones. I doubt that he would have felt that my silent reference to Superman was particularly humorous.

I said, "I'm just a wannabe veterinarian but I'm pretty sure that your shoulder is dislocated. I think that is a much better option than a fractured scapula or humerus, however."

We sat there contemplating his fate for a minute or so and he said, "Is there something we can do about it?"

This was before the days of satellite cell phones. I had a radio to communicate with fire lookouts but it only worked if I was located on a ridgetop, not down deep in a valley. I said, "We could possibly have a float plane land on the lake or get an army helicopter in but it would take at least half a day to make all the arrangements. If you are willing, it seems like it's worth a try to put your shoulder back in place." It seemed like he started sweating again at that prospect. I was pretty sure that the ball on the end of the humerus had been shoved forward out of the socket in the scapula. It seemed like a fairly simple mechanical process to put it back in place if you could forget how much it was going to hurt.

I could almost hear the worry gears in his brain grinding and was pretty sure I could see the beads of sweat begin to reform on his forehead but he said, "It looks like I have nothing to lose."

I said, "Here is my plan." If I put a roll of material in your armpit to act as a leverage point and I push your elbow in towards your rib cage this might lever the ball free and let it slide back into the socket. Easy. Peasy." Now he was really sweating.

We put his injured arm and head through the neck hole of his T-shirt. By incorporating more fabric in the rolled-up tail of his T-shirt we created a lever to be placed in his armpit.

I told him that on the count of THREE I was going to press his elbow firmly against his rib cage. He nodded grimly in agreement and we were ready to proceed. I started counting and on the count of TWO forced the elbow in. There was a shriek and I'm pretty sure some birds flew out of a nearby tree. I had pushed with my right hand but I had my left hand steadying the shoulder and I felt the socket return to its normal configuration. He said some choice words that wouldn't be recommended for little children's big ears.

Success! We sat for a minute in silence and then I remembered that my dinner had been cooking. The potatoes carefully wrapped in foil and tucked into the coals at the edge of the fire had turned into charcoal briquettes. The cornbread baking in the Dutch oven had become a blackened miniature flying saucer. The yellow jackets were attempting to carry away my chuck steak which fortunately I had not yet placed on the grill. I guess that in those moments there had been *bigger fish to fry*.

What a sense of euphoria settled in and around my camp! We were suddenly aware of the sounds of Spinola Creek gurgling nearby, some Stellar Jays squawking in the trees, and my horses nickering hungrily from their corral because I had forgotten to give them their pellets. I was also starved but dinner was pretty much beyond rescue or repair.

While my friend sat in my camp chair with a stunned look on his face, I salvaged the remanence of my chuck steak from the yellow jackets and chopped it into small bits which I stir-fried in my cast iron frying pan with some onion. I had some chicken noodle soup and when I added the steak bits, some more water, and some spaghetti, I had created something unique that vaguely resembled a dinner meal for the two of us. If you are hungry enough out in the woods almost anything tastes good. Besides, chicken soup is supposed to have magical healing properties as well. Some Oreo cookies helped to mask the strange flavors of the main course.

After dinner for us and the horses, I saddled up my horse and rode in the dark back to his campsite to retrieve his pack. This was long before the era of LED headlamps and the D cells in my government issue headlamp had died and corroded into their container. My tent frame had two canvas cots so after dinner we finished off a cold Olympia Beer, a few more of the Oreo cookies, and four aspirin for him and snuggled into our sleeping bags. I slept like a log but I suspect he slept rather fitfully.

The situation looked even better the next morning but he was pretty sore and decided he would just spend the day in my camp. I rode out with my horse and pack animals to finish the work started the previous day. By mid-afternoon I was back at my camp and we decided to see if we could get him out to the trailhead and his car. He couldn't carry his pack so I saddled up my personal horse and put him on board. I tacked up one of the pack horses to carry his backpack and scrambling on board the other pack horse bareback. Then I led my four-legged, two eared, long nosed, one tailed ambulance down the trail to Salmon La Sac. The horses thought they were going home so the miles passed quickly and uneventfully. Three hours later I waved goodbye as he drove down the road towards home in Seattle. But by then it was dark and I had no food and only the light jacket I had tied on behind my saddle. The horses were reluctant and more than a little disappointed when I turned them back up the trail to return to my camp. I couldn't see a thing but horses have amazing vision even in total darkness. I must have dozed off part of the way because it certainly didn't seem like three and a half hours of hours of riding before I heard the clip clopping of their shod feet on the wooden deck of the footbridge. I unsaddled, watered, and brushed them and put them back in their corral with an extra ration of pellets for their effort. I drank a big dipper of cold stream water, finished off the last of Oreo the cookies and at an unknown hour went to bed. *Moments later,* when the sun woke me in the morning I got up in my long john's and watered and fed the horses and then collapsed back in bed for a three-hour morning nap. When I awoke at lunch time, I didn't feel guilty at all and decided to have breakfast. 16 hot cakes, 4 eggs, half a pound of bacon, some fried potatoes, buttered fried bread, and two mugs of hot chocolate almost satisfied me. Then I saddled the horses and tried to complete a day's worth of my usual work.

I never did hear from my unnamed friend but nevertheless look back at the experience and feel that we shared a bond that neither of us will ever forget.

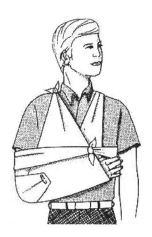

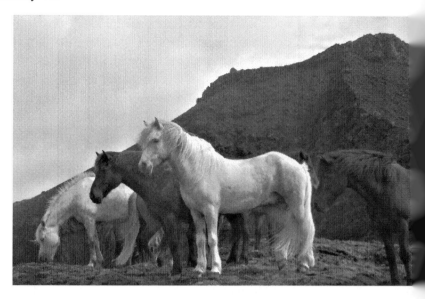

THE ICELANDIC HORSE

Horses (similar to Norwegian Fjords) were first carried by ship across the North Atlantic to Iceland in the 9th and 10th centuries by Norse settlers who left Scandinavia because of civil strife and shortage of arable land. Later settlers to the Northern British Isles also brought horses which would develop into the Shetland, Highland, and Connemara ponies. In 982 the Icelandic Parliament (one of the world's oldest democracies) passed laws prohibiting the importation of additional horses so the breed has been pure for more than 1000 years. This policy continues to this day. The modern Icelandic horse has similar DNA to Faeroe pony, Yakut pony, Nordlandshest of Norway, Norwegian Fjord horse, and Mongolian horse.

There were early periods of selective breeding for color and conformation, but volcanic eruptions in 1783 to 1784 and periods of severe climate (mini ice ages) caused the loss of up to 70% of the horse population but also selected for the hardiest horses. The first Icelandic breed societies were established in 1904 and the first registry in 1923. Some were exported to Great Britain in the early 1900's for coal mine ponies and in the 1940's some went to Germany. There are now 80,000 Icelandic horses in Iceland with a human population of 330,000 (1 horse for every 4 people), and 100,000 Icelandics elsewhere in the world (mainly Germany).

Historically horses were used for sheep herding, transportation, human food, racing and showing. When traveling by land, a horseman would bring extra horses along in a herd with 3 or 4 horses per rider. A family taking their sheep back to mountain pasture in the spring would lead a string of pack horses tied head to tail along with a herd of loose horses. Riders in front and behind kept the loose herd organized and under control. There were few parasite or diseases and the horse's natural hardiness made them the perfect animal for the early Icelandic people.

Icelandic horses are small weighing 725 to 850 lbs. (330 to 385 kilos in Icelandic) and are 13 to 14 hands tall. A hand is four inches. You'll have to do the math. They come in all colors and color patterns except perhaps appaloosa and overo paint. Solid blacks, browns, sorrels, grays and whites predominate. It is said that they have all the colors found in a basic Crayola box. Line back buckskins (or duns) have zebra stripes on their upper forelegs and a black line down the middle of their back that continues into their mane creating a black part in the middle with tan hair on either side. The crest of their neck is thick and wide to accommodate all this mane. Their bushy mane and forelock makes you think of a Dr. Seuss character and it is so thick that only the tips of the ears show and the eyes are partially hidden behind the forelock. Since riders cue on horse's ears and eyes it takes a little longer to get to appreciate their friendly willing personality. Their long low-set full tail may almost drag on the ground.

They are long lived and used well into their late 20's but being slow maturing they are not heavily used before they are 6 years old. One reached an age of 56. They are very hardy with few diseases or parasites. In the winter an Icelandic horse seems twice as big due to their heavy double winter coat which can even keep snow on their back from melting. They are surprisingly uniform in size and shape with almost all wearing the same shoe sizes (00 or 000 typically hardened with borium on the toe and heals) and with similar girth sizes. Some, however, are bred for work or as pack animals and are more heavily built. Eyes are large, soft, and wide set if you can find them under the forelock. Perhaps because there are no predators in Iceland Icelandic horses are not easily spooked and are easy to handle and be around. Herdsmen comfortably walk amongst a tightly pack herd of horses to catch the one they want without fear of being kicked.

They are most commonly kept in herds and thus show characteristic unseen with our smaller groups of horses. Foals do rear and play but kicking is infrequent. They might threaten but the threatened horse quickly backs away avoiding a confrontation. There are obvious dominant horses within the herd but bite marks are rarely visible. Many have a best friend and the two are always seen together if conditions allow. They swat each other's flies and *nag* each other's backs. If things get really tense, rather than killing each other, horses sometimes squat rump to rump pushing backwards into each other while squealing. On narrow trails they quickly fall into single file in a relatively prearranged order with obvious leaders, followers, and trailers. It is interesting to observe that when traveling as a herd they often walk to the same audible rhythm like an equine marching band with simultaneous clip clops. The leaders seem to find the best places to put their feet and the followers travel more securely placing their feet in the same place. They sometimes even follow almost blindly with their head buried in the tail of the horse ahead while at the same time never seeming to stumble.

Watching their moving feet can be fascinating. Lava flows can have truly nasty leg breaking holes in the surface but Icelandics travel through this terrain never missing a stride. Some have a very high natural leg lift befitting a gaited horse show ring setting. Some have an under-stride like a Paso Fino. Some walk like a quarter horse with back feet over placing the front feet, and some move like a Tennessee Walker with a moderate over-stride. Almost all tolt (also spelled toelt) with a distinct 4 beat rhythm leaving one foot on the ground resulting in a smooth ride. (In a trot the whole horse is in the air jolting the rider when all the weight hits the ground). The more even and distinct the 1, 2, 3, 4 count is the smoother the ride. Some are pacy with both legs on one side rising and landing simultaneously kind of like the drive arms on a steam locomotive. This results in a hard side to side motion rough on the rider but capable of 30 mph speeds. A smooth tolting horse leaves the riders head, neck, shoulders, and torso almost stationary with only the waist and buttocks rocking rhythmically from side to side. A rough tolting horse is like a trot but a little smoother due to the shorter stride.

Tack is simple. English hunt seat saddles seem almost universal giving the horse maximum freedom of shoulder movement. Icelandics have amazingly similar low withers so the saddle gullets were relatively shallow. Rain gear is attached behind the cantle with roller buckle leather straps. Pads or blankets are not used in Iceland. I don't know why. The fact that the island gets 200 inches of rain may be a factor because blankets would always be wet. They are a little thicker skinned and their dense hair coat also protects. White haired scald marks are not observed on horse's backs vouching for the fact that pads are not a necessity. Broken bits also seem to be universal from a simple D ring snaffle to a broken curb bit with a leather or chain curb piece. Cavessans are universal helping to keep the bit centered and engaged in the horse's mouth.

Hardy, willing, forward going, sturdy, friendly, trusting, adaptable, easy keepers, durable, sociable.

WHAT'S NOT TO LIKE ABOUT AN ICELANDIC HORSE?

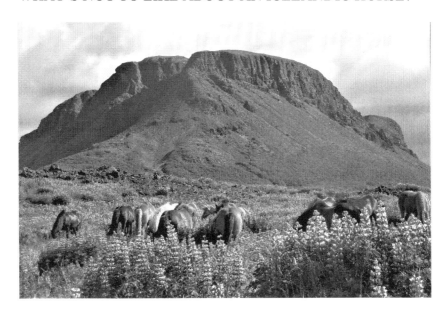

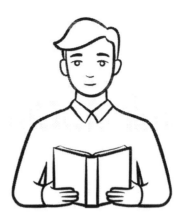

ON BEING A STUDENT

Student status is at best an imperfect condition. Countless hours are spent learning endless quantities of information but educators have historically not necessarily communicated how to use and integrate that information in practice. Such is the plight of a veterinary student. You study animal anatomy at a gross and microscopic level and learn about disease causing agents or physical events that can cause injury.

When it's all said and done you may have a long list of things that can happen but little concept of the frequency and likelihood that they would actually occur. During your senior year of veterinary school, you start your clinical rotations and actually work with animals and learn to diagnose and treat their problems. WSU had a herd of Holstein Friesian dairy cows so animal science students could learn about the dairy industry. The black and white cows provided delicious ice cream through the university outlet store called Ferdinand's Ice Cream Shoppe and also produced region wide famous Cougar Gold cheese. (Does Shoppe seem a little pretentious for a cow college?) The herd also provided table milk for university student dining halls. There was also an opportunity for veterinary students to work with dairy cows when doing large animal clinic rotations. We visited the herd once or twice a week to observe normal cows as well as work with any disease or health issues.

On one occasion when our small group of students visited the herd accompanied by our professor Dr. *Andy* Anderson, the herdsman said, "You might want to check that cow over there. She's calving but seems to be taking longer than usual."

Our instructor let us scrub up and reach into the birth canal to determine if there was any kind of problem with the calving process.

The first student said, "I can feel the head and two front feet but something doesn't seem right."

The next two students reached in and they all agreed with one commenting, "The head seems upside down."

I was the last person to check the cow and was therefore under no time pressure because there was no one else waiting for their turn. I had thought about what the first student said, and when I began my examination, I found the head and *four* feet. A calf normally delivers as if it were diving into water. When you think of the shape of front legs versus back legs it's fairly easy to determine one from the other based on the shape of the joints. I decided that all four feet and the head were in an upside-down position.

Considering this I said, "I think this is a shistosoma circumflexus calf."

The professor looked at me and tried to hide the slight superior smirk on his face and said, "That almost never happens. Even I have never seen one. It can't be that. It's just twins."

We were out of time so we loaded into the university van for the trip back to the vet school campus.

Shisto means split and circumflexis means bent backwards and inverted. Sadly, but very rarely, the belly wall of a fetus does not develop. Imagine no muscles or skin where your belly button is. The back muscles nevertheless contract but there are no muscles to counteract this force so the fetus is bent backwards like doing a back bend. This would result in the head and front legs as well as the back legs being rotated in the wrong direction. Mother nature had mistakenly created a non-viable contortionist calf.

A few days later I happen to encounter Dr. Anderson as we were finishing up our rounds in the large animal barn. He said, "I'm sure you remember that Holstein cow from last week."

I said. "Yes! I remember her. What was the outcome?

He said, "The herdsman called me later that evening and said that the cow had not calved and asked if I would come out and examine her. The examination was certainly confusing with body parts in strange locations and positions. We ultimately decided to do a C-section since there seemed to be no way to deliver the calf normally. I want to give you credit for being correct. It was an abnormal calf exactly as you had diagnosed, a shistosomas circumflexis. I have been doing this for over 30 years and never seen one. I guess you're never too old to learn. I am sure that you know this is an exceedingly rare condition and you and I are in a very selective group even to have diagnosed and seen one. You might want to know that the cow is doing fine and is one of their best milkers."

These calves have abnormal circulation and not having a proper diaphragm are unable to breathe and thus die almost immediately after they are delivered and have lost their umbilical lifeline.

During my career as a veterinarian I have seen cyclopia calves with only one abnormal eye in the middle of the forehead, 5 legged calves with the fifth leg attached like a small branch below the elbow, two-headed calves with the deformed second head attached at the neck like a headhunter's trophy, spinal bifida where the spinal cord only extends two-thirds of the way down the back, cleft palate where the hard palate is not formed and closed, and arthrogryposis where are joints are effectively frozen because something prevented the fetus from swimming and moving while in the uterus. Sadly, but fortunately, these mistakes of nature have other defects incompatible with life and are either born dead or survive for only a few minutes.

The veterinary school curriculum, has become too large to assimilate and gain proficiency in a four-year course. A year's internship would benefit the industry with more qualified new graduates but would also increase the cost of an already expensive education. Human medicine utilizes physician assistants to great advantage. Much of a veterinarian's work is fairly routine and could be delegated to a trained and licensed veterinary assistant.

I WONDER WHERE ALL THE BIRDIES IS

My yard has been invaded by marauding multitudes of migrating snowbird American Robbins returning from their winter sojourn in southern climes. There must have been at least 60 with more awaiting their turn from the nearby trees. I guess they had to take a number. They woke me too early this Sunday morning with their annoying little chirps and glaringly bright orange/red breasts as they flitted and hopped around in my sun filling backyard. How totally annoying!

The poor little innocent bugses and wormses didn't stand a chance. You could almost hear the crunch and squish as their writhing little bug bodies were crushed between the bird's ruthless black greedy little beaks. Form a mental image of the poor slimy dirty little worms screaming as their limbs and heads were torn from their bodies and they were wrenched from their secure homes in the dark sandy loam outside my window. Imagine the bird's Adam's Apples contracting and convulsing as this now unrecognizable material was forced down into the depths of their mysterious digestive system.

The obnoxious cock Robbins were chasing after the more modest lady Robbins who were trying to ignore the annoying dog whistles and chirps. I suspect the boys were only thinking about mating. Did I hear some appropriate complaining squawks reminiscent of the Me-too Movement from the ladies? The little blighters occasionally stopped and cocked their head sideways with a haughty knowing little smirk on their faces. Then with an arrogant little flick of their tail, they moved on.

When some unheard sound or motion startled them, they arose as one and deposited several dribbling splats of a gray white material on my windows. Now I'll either have to wash the windows or hope for a rainstorm to do it for me. Who wants to view the world through gray-colored glasses? However, they soon returned and continued marching as a *company front* across my lawn like marauding army ants. The poor little shoots of fragile delicate new grass were being trampled down by dirty little feet just as they were struggling to break into the sunlight.

After reconsidering my curmudgeonly grumpiness, I said to myself. "I do hope the birds will stay a while. Maybe I should invite some to spend the summer here with me in my backyard."

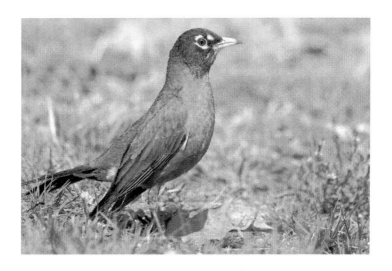

THE CUBAN HORSE

An Easter 2016 People to People adventure to Cuba prompted me to observe, research, and write this brief study on the Cuban horse. As of July 2019, such trips are no longer possible due to a travel ban imposed by our president.

In 1494 when Columbus made his second voyage to the new world, he brought pigs, cattle, and horses. (Maybe chickens and probably rats.) Horses were eventually carried to Cuba where a breeding facility was established. As Italian, Portuguese, and Spanish explorers came and went some horses escaped or were abandoned. Direct descendants of these Iberian breeds still exist in the island nation of Cuba. The horses are grouped collectively as Criollo and most originate from Spanish horses brought to Cuba in 1751 by Diego Velázquez. They strongly resemble the modern Paso Fino or Peruvian Paso breeds and many have a dark line down their back and zebra like stripes on their upper legs. Small by modern US standards, 700 - 800 pounds, 13 1/2 - 14 1/2 hands, tending toward darker colors, narrow but deep chested, large soft eyes, refined head, and with feet slightly larger than would be expected for a horse of that size.

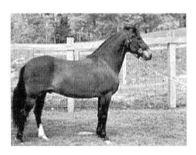

Today there are about 1,000,000 horses and additionally a total of 300,000 cattle, mules, and donkeys. The Cuban government, beginning in the 1960's, established breeding farms and a registry for the Cuban Paso Fino which is a gaited breed noted for its fast smooth walk. There may only be 500 to 800 in existence. Other breeds are the Cuban Pinto resulting from crossing the Criollo horses with Quarter Horses and Thoroughbreds which can be tobiano or overo, the Cuban Trotter which is a Criollo horse crossed with Canadian trotters, and the Patibarcino which is a Criollo crossed with an Andalusian or Barb horse which usually has blue, slate or silver dun coloring.

In the 1950's Cuba was ruled by the corrupt dictator Fuglencia Batista who was supported by the US government. Fidel Castro, his brother Raul, and Argentinian doctor Che Guevara led what is known as the 26th of July Movement that overthrew Batista on 1 January 1959. Many felt the rebellion would fail and left Cuba thinking that the departure would be temporary and they could soon return. They left everything only to have it soon nationalized by the new government. In 1960 in a tit for tat retaliation all US businesses in Cuba were nationalized and President Kennedy initiated the US embargo of trade with Cuba. When no one would assist him in developing the Cuban economy, Castro turned to the USSR which was only too happy to establish a military economic presence in backyard of the US. This was followed by the abortive Bay of Pigs Invasion, the Cuban missile crisis, and the collapse of the USSR in 1991.

The post USSR time is known as the *special period* in Cuba and it continues to this day. The Soviet Union had trade agreements with Cuba whereby they supplied some of the food, machinery, and almost all of the petroleum. When the Russians pulled out, Cuba lost 80% of its imports and exports, 35% of GDP, and oil imports fell to 10% of its pre-1990 level. Cuba's industry, transportation and agriculture collapsed in the absence of industrial petroleum products. Food rationing began, power outages were common, bus waits could be 3 hours, and the average Cuban lost 20lbs.

Showing amazing resilience, the Cubans survived albeit somewhat marginally. Australian aid and technology arrived especially in agriculture with raised garden beds, rooftop gardens, and community gardens wherever there was vacant urban space. Transportation was improvised with semi-trucks converted to 300 passenger people haulers, box trucks converted to buses, importation of 1.5 million Chinese bicycles which promptly fell apart, and resurrection of late 1950's Chevrolet cars (still seen in large numbers on urban Cuban streets). Almost everything was, and is, owned by the state including the vintage cars. Food is subsidized but you must have a ration card, everyone is guaranteed a government job if they want it, and free education and medicine is available for everyone. Everyone travels with a shopping bag in hope that they might pass a government store and discover that a scarce item was in stock. It could sell out in minutes. There is one MD for every 25 families. However, wages in government jobs are $20 - $40 per month but it takes $360 for a family of four. Consequently, both parents work as perhaps do older children and outside private sources of income must be arranged. Anything the people can produce locally from handicrafts to home grown food is available almost everywhere. Even trash has value and none is left in the streets. The absence of fast food also keeps the streets clean as do countless street dogs. Recently Cuba had 1 million tourists from mainly Europe and Canada providing desperately needed foreign exchange to purchase technology, oil, and machinery. Cuba has traded doctors and medical technology to Venezuela for oil. The economic crisis beginning in 2015 in Venezuela has put Cuba in a major bind as the US embargos the Venezuelan dictator and anyone who deals with him economically.

All this has led to the resurrection of the utilitarian horse in Cuba. They are not a luxury item but rather a means to earn an income and feed a family for the lower income members of the Cuban population. Most cannot afford a motorized vehicle so the horses fill that position in the national economy. Some Cubans say, "There are those who walk, and those who ride. Thanks be to God, we ride."

Horses seem to be ubiquitous with about one horse for every 12 people and all of them serving a useful purpose. (In contrast in the US there is about one horse for every 110 people with a much lower utilization efficiency). Horses are staked out everywhere there is grass, often only by a halter rope and still saddled or harnessed. Roadside ditches, fences, trees, bushes, rocks, and old tires all serve. Most are used to pull light carts or wagons in a single hitch at a trot while a few are under saddle moving at a running walk like a paso. They compete at 6mph wearing blinkers with bus traffic going 60mph on provincial highways and must obey all traffic laws. Looking down a smaller city street you might see 8 or 10 carts hauling people or goods with horses in fact outnumbered automobiles. They cost $250 to $300. Surely there must be animal/auto collisions but I saw the carriages causing no traffic problems. Perhaps this is due to the fact that horses are a way of life in Cuba and automobile drivers are more educated and considerate. Our bus made frequent hard stops to avoid a lone small horse pulling a two or four wheeled cart down a highway.

Many of the cart horses were well mannered stallions but this wasn't for financial reasons since veterinary services were free including vaccinations and deworming. Urban cart horses had poop catchers suspended from the shafts and there was no manure in the streets. Country roads were a little more fertilized. All horses were shod with most having tow clips on the shoes. Occasionally you could hear a shoe jingle indicating the need to be reset. City tourist carriage horses seemed to have adequate foot care but this did not seem to be the case in more rural areas. Horse shoes and farriers cost money. They seemed amazingly universally docile and willingly shifting from a walk to a trot with a vocal click.

Operating a city carriage required a license and necessitated 4 horses: one for the morning, one for the afternoon, and two resting at home. At the end of the day the operator drove or rode one horse home leading the other. Little hay was available and apparently no grain with the horses managing solely on pasture. Most were lean but not poor. My fellow travelers pointed out poor horses to me wanting my comment but I felt most were aged. Horse meat is eaten since there is a general shortage of protein. It is illegal to eat a cow without government permission with a significant fine. The horses were not heavy enough for farm labor and oxen teams were frequently seen plowing small fields due to the tractor shortage.

Carts came in all forms from two wheeled to four wheeled, tires of steel, hard rubber, bicycle rubber or even automotive, sprung or unsprung, fancy or plain, covered or open, and carrying from two to the legal maximum of 8 passengers. There is no exchange money to buy carts on the world market so they must construct and improvise locally with no two carts being the same. Some had an automotive battery to power a boom box and many allowed bicyclists to be towed behind.

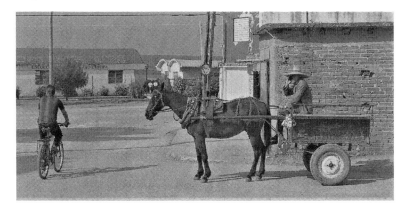

Temperature was in the low to mid 90's and it was an issue for the horses. Their thin skin and short hair coat seemed to help and none seemed to sweat profusely. However, when at rest they breathed heavily to assist in cooling. Little shade was available. I sensed that the horse is a very important part of the Cuban economy and also a prized family possession helping a family to survive and provide for itself. That said, money is short and it showed in ill-fitting equipment, relatively poor body condition, and marginal foot care. I think the people did the best they could with what they had.

There are numerous animal aid associations, most funded by Cuban Americans, attempting to assist in the health and welfare of Cuban dogs and horses. Their lobbying has finally yielded results because, beginning in 2018, animal welfare laws are being developed.

Cuba is a strange juxtaposition of modern medicine and technology awaiting financing and development against a barter/trade/ subsistence existence. The people seem resolute, frustrated, and eagerly await the better times they see in the future.

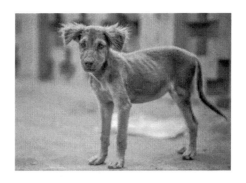

CUBAN DOGS

During this 2016 spring tour of Cuba we used a large motorsailer as a floating mobile hotel. The boat sailed and motored around the periphery of the island nation and we went ashore every day to visit cities and points of political or historical interest. We were closely watched and attended by our mandatory Cuban guide but she was understandably reluctant to talk about economic, social, or political issues. Our Cuban American tour guide was better informed and also able to help us understand the economic and political plight of the Cuban citizens.

There were dogs everywhere. Most were smallish, wiry, and long-legged with a short light-colored hair coat. During the heat of the day they would lie stretched out in a dusty secluded shady spot but get up occasionally to follow the shade as the sun traversed the sky. In the cool of the morning or evening you could see them trotting around purposefully perhaps looking for handouts or just socializing. If you listened carefully in the evening you could always hear a dog barking somewhere. I suspect that these were the dogs that actually had a home and a fenced-in yard and they were the fulfilling their role as a watchdog and natural alarm system.

The national dog of Cuba is the Havanese which is a member of the Bichon family of dogs. These dogs share some common characteristics such as a tail that curls up over the back, a short muzzle and slightly droopy ears. They have a long silky or curly hair without any undercoat. Thus, while their hair is pretty and helps to keep them cool it makes them cold intolerant. They are very friendly happy bouncy dogs that are likely to attach themselves to one person and are thus sometimes called Velcro dogs. They seem to be the prized possession of the wealthier Cubans and are obviously spoiled and often seen sporting colorful doggie sweaters and rhinestone studded collars. There was a good chance they would be carried around by their owners and certainly were not traveling around free and unattached.

Medicine and care for the Cuban *people* is free but the 8,000 or so Cuban veterinarians are paid the typical $15 to $30 government salary and almost all of their work is directed towards agriculture and food-producing animals. There are very few private veterinary clinics and only the wealthy can afford to take their valued pets there for treatment. Services and supplies run in the $5 to $20 range but a Cuban citizen only gets the government salary. Because human healthcare, food, utilities, and transportation are free or subsidized, Cuba is actually one of the more economically healthy countries of Central America.

The semi-feral street dogs were much less fortunate. Dogs are only moderately self-sufficient and, in some way, depend on humans for survival. Some apparently had owners for they had collars and tags indicating they had been vaccinated at least for rabies. Most were timid and shy but sometimes showed a little courage in the presence of strangers or tourists. If you sat quietly, they would cautiously approach with their tail and head down in a submissive posture hoping for some sort of food hand out. They appeared to have a territory or neighborhood for they appeared at the same locations on successive days. Once it was fully dark the dogs disappeared from the streets and must have had some sort of a home or shelter at an unknown location. Neutering was an unaffordable luxury for most people as was evidenced by the presence of many puppies. There are government animal control policies and if animals become too numerous and a problem at a location, they will be held briefly for a possible owner to claim. If not claimed they are rather inhumanely euthanized using poisoned food.

Cats were present but less evident. Finca Vigia was the home of Ernest Hemingway when he lived in Cuba. It is now a museum and we were told by the curator that the cats there were direct descendants of those owned by this great author. Cats are less expensive to feed and can supplement their diet by hunting rodents and birds. Overeating and obesity were certainly not a problem for either cats or dogs.

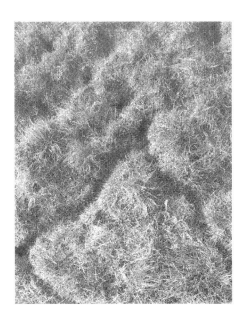

MY BACKYARD

After the snow finally melted off, I courageously determined to tour and inspect my backyard domain. Other than to restock my birdy feeders, I hadn't really ventured outside the comfort of my man cave for months. The fireplace, hot chocolate, and NETFLIX had been overly addictive. I put on my Elmer Fudd hat, my camouflage quilted Carhartt coat, my long wool stockings, my insulated Redwing boots, and loosened up my telescoping walking staff. I wanted to be prepared for anything.

Boldly stepping off my concrete sidewalk onto the dangerous grassy unknown, I was confronted by a most terrifying sight. Under the cover of the winter snow blanket there had been ground level warfare going on. After the warm days and Chinook wind had melted the snow, I could see that there were foxholes and trenches and tunnels everywhere. Foot paths radiated from the huge holes like the streets of Paris from the Arc de Triomphe. The open trenches must have been created by mini Kubota excavators. Some tunnels disappeared deep underground like miniature Elon Musk hyperloop tunnels while others were close to the surface as if they had been bored by miniature water seeking Sandworms as in Frank Herbert's science fiction novel "Dune".

What had caused this devastation? I feared that if I ventured out into this dreadful wasteland, I might be drawn screaming down into an underground warren of tunnels never to be seen again. And then I saw the perpetrator of this holocaust. It poked its nasty little head and bulky shoulders out of one of the larger holes and stared at me nearsightedly with a sickeningly evil grin. The dirty little bugger had gray brown dense hair, short round ears, squat little legs, dark sneaky beady little eyes, short brown twitching whiskers, and a fat stumpy runt of a tail. Its teeth and claws were even more frightening. They were long, yellowed, and obviously dangerously sharp. Was there a stringy glob of green drool hanging from its chin?

Fearing for my life and sanity, I rushed back inside and slammed and triple locked the door securely behind me. After catching my breath and letting my pulse return to normal, I changed back in into my fuzzy green pajamas with the string tie waist, blue bunny rabbit slippers, and white terry cloth bathrobe and sat down at the computer to research this dreadful invader. Surely some misinformation could be found on Facebook or Twitter?

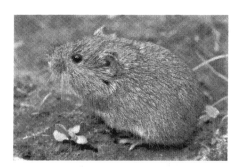

The vole, or field mouse, is a small burrow dwelling rodent often mistaken for a mouse or gopher although it is related to mice, lemmings, and muskrats. Compared to a mouse, it is plumper, about 4 inches long, has smaller round ears, smaller eyes, a shorter blunt nose, a short fur covered tail and beaver like incisors for chewing roots and grasses. It can have 5 to 10 litters per year with 5 to 10 pups per litter. They reach sexual maturity in one month and have a gestation period of just three weeks. Using Watson, my personal pocket supercomputer, I have calculated that with full litters and 100% survival, two voles could potentially produce 170,000 offspring in six months. Surely Watson is in error?

Fortunately, a vole's life expectancy is only about six months but a pair can nevertheless typically produce 100 descendants each year. Mother nature has also conveniently introduced about 90% mortality in the first month of life. Under ideal conditions imagine how quickly they could populate and rule the earth. Next year's blockbuster movie could be "Planet of the Voles".

They are mainly herbivores and primarily eat grass and above ground forage. However, when they tunnel, they eat plant roots and grass rhizomes and can even kill small trees and shrubs by girdling them or chewing off all the smaller water siphoning adventitious roots. They can be devastating to hay and legume crops taking as much as 30% of the production and reaching numbers as high as 4000 voles per acre. They, like mice, are also opportunists and will eat insects, dead animal matter, seeds, and nuts if the opportunity arises.

On occasion I have carefully watered, fertilized, and weeded my garden root vegetables with the expectation of a bountiful harvest in the fall. When I pulled the beets or carrots by their tops out of the ground, I discovered that the vole from his underground hideaway had traveled along the same row and carefully eaten away almost everything that was below ground. In two days, a large onion and even its large green top disappeared. I trust the vole family had breath freshener in its underground family room. I have seen healthy-looking bean shoots be snatched and disappear underground right before my eyes. Where is Jack with his magic bean seeds when you need him?

Predators are helpful but actually have little impact on vole population. Poisons have variable benefit but also pose risk to other species and ecosystems. There are safe products used by commercial orchards, however. Early cold in the winter before snowfall, can freeze the ground and put a limit on winter breeding, but sometimes you just have to get out of the way and let nature do its thing.

For the animals that can't migrate to more temperate climes winter can be harsh time struggling to survive. By January the ground is covered by a frozen sheet of ice and snow, but beneath the protective crust the voles are creating extensive tunnel highways through the dry dead grass. If the ground is unfrozen, they make shallow tunnels in the top few inches of dirt as well. They must feel secure and complacent in their quiet winter world.

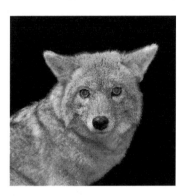

At this time of year, the coyote hunts both day and night. The family sing-a-longs are absent as each animal tries independently to make it through the winter. Absent too are the playful games of chase played by the young pups at the den entrance. Watching them hunt for voles is a fascinating pastime. They travel across the wind hoping to pick up the tantalizing scent of their next meal. Then they stop and listen intently, perhaps hearing the voles scrambling through their tunnels beneath the snow crust. Sensing an animal below, the coyote springs almost straight up into the air and pounces down stiff legged with all four paws collapsing the snow or ice tunnel roof over the vole. A second jump avalanches the tunnel behind the vole and after a few seconds of frantic digging the coyote is rewarded with a tasty morsel.

One short winter afternoon as dark storm clouds approached from west, I observed a young coyote hunting in my pasture. He was ignored by the nearby horses pawing through the snow for grass and who seemed to realize he posed no threat to them. I watched, with a cup of hot chocolate in my hand, with binoculars through my living room window for about an hour. In that time, he caught and ate 5 voles, peed on a low scrub, and trotted off to the west towards his winter den. I guess there was no *catch and release* policy in effect at that time.

In summer when the horses have chewed the grass down short in some areas, Great Blue Herons stop in for afternoon meals. With their long legs and bills nature designed them to feed on frogs, amphibians, and small fish in shallow waters. Undaunted by the lack of water they sweep in like avian B-52 bombers and with an awkward hop or two come to rest in the middle of my pasture. Like Chinese tai chi exercisers, they move in extreme slow motion and proceed across my field waiting for a vole to foolishly expose himself from his hole. With a lightning-fast stab of the beak they grab the hapless little critter and carry him to an area where the grass is short. They drop him on the ground and if he moves, they bap him on the head a few more times until he stops moving. Then they pick him up, flipping him so that he can swallowed down head-first with one gulp. Then the whole slow-motion dance and eating routine begins again. They catch and eat five or six voles per hour.

When I am irrigating my horse pasture in the summer, my border collie Piper comes along to help and supervise. Just like a coyote, she travels at right angles to the breeze and if she picks up a scent she stops and turns her body in that direction. Then she freezes with only her ears twitching and waits, watches, listens, and smells. If she seems convinced there is a vole in the grass, she springs straight up in the air and tries to pounce on the unlucky rodent. She usually has a success rate of 50 or 60% and when we get back to the house, I can congratulate her on having hunted and exterminated her daily catch limit of voles

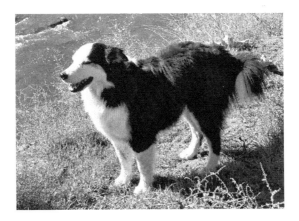

When Piper was a pampered perky pretty playful pup and was learning how to hunt hairy hole-hiding hapless heathen herbivores, she would catch them and turn them loose again to play with them. If they failed to move, she would growl impatiently at them. On a few occasions, if she got too close, they would latch onto her nose or lip and the growl would quickly become a yipe. She, unlike some humans, learned from her mistake and hasn't made that error again

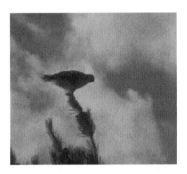

I have Red Tailed Hawks, Cooper's Hawks, Northern goshawks, Rough-legged, and Sharp-shinned Hawks as well as Short-eared and Barn Owls that like to perch in the leader branches of my Austrian Pine windbreak trees. They watch patiently until they see some movement far beyond the reach of human vision and then glide down to capture a vole or occasional young rabbit or quail. Birds of prey have better color vision, (more cones in their retina), greater visual acuity, (more rods in their retina), and the center portion of their retina also magnifies the image like a telephoto lens thus giving them truly remarkable distance vision. They have the equivalent of 20/5 vision or see at 20 feet what we see at 5 feet.

When I have to look at my face in the mirror in the morning, I am glad I don't have hawk-like vision.

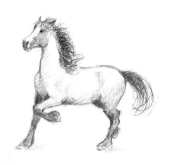

TENNESSEE STUD

Back about eighteen and twenty-five
I left Tennessee very much alive
I never would've made it through the Arkansas
mud
If I hadn't been riding on the Tennessee Stud

Had some trouble with my sweetheart's Pa
One of her brothers was a bad outlaw
I wrote a letter to my Uncle Fud
And I rode away on the Tennessee Stud

The Tennessee Stud was long and lean
The color of the sun and his eyes were green
He had the nerve and he had the blood
There never was a horse like Tennessee Stud

Drifted on down into no man's land
I crossed the river called the Rio Grande

Raced my horse with the Spaniard's bold
Til I got me a skin full of silver and gold

Me and the gambler, we couldn't agree
We got in a fight over Tennessee
Pulled our guns and he fell with a thud
And I rode away on the Tennessee Stud

The Tennessee Stud was long and lean
The color of the sun and his eyes were green
He had the nerve and he had the blood
There was never a horse like the Tennessee Stud

I rode right back across Arkansas
I whipped her brother and
I whipped her Pa
I found that girl with the golden hair
She was riding on a Tennessee Mare

Pretty little baby on the cabin floor
Little horse colt playing 'round the door
I love the girl with the golden hair
And the Tennessee Stud loves the Tennessee Mare

The Tennessee Stud was long and lean
The color of the sun and his eyes were green
He had the nerve and he had the blood
There was never a horse like the Tennessee Stud

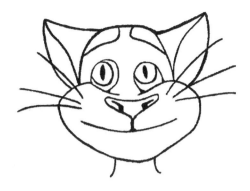

TOMMY THE BARN CAT

To the tune of "Frosty the Snowman"

Tommy the barn cat,
Was a crabby noisy sole.
With a long black tail,
A white mustache,
And two eyes as black as coal.

He'll dance all around,
Till you put sardines in his dish.
And if you wake up,
With him on your chest,
His breath will smell like fish

CHORUS

There must have been some Siamese in,
That old black cat they'd found.
For when they put him out the door,
He began to yowl around.

He'll hunt all night,
And leave mouse guts on your floor.
But he'll make a fuss,
And he can surely cuss,
When you kick him out the door.

He'll sleep all day,
And leave fur balls on your bed.
With a cough and wheeze,
And a "Pardon me please,"
It'll make your eyes see red.

CHORUS

He surely thought of you that day,
When he brought the rat inside.
Cus when he dropped it on the floor,
Your eyes were open wide.

Yes, Tommy the barn cat.
Brings you joy every day.
When he disappears,
You need have no fears.
He'll be back again someday.

Oh, Tommy the barn cat,
Knows when he has made a score.
Cause he's got nine lives.,
And you realize,
He'll be 'round forever more.

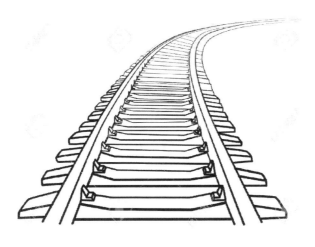

16 TONS

For the railroads to progress across the northwestern United States frontier, a number of factors had to come together. Land or a right-of-way, fill and ballast to construct the roadbed, timber for railroad ties, steel for the rails, manpower to put all this together, and finally coal to fuel the steam engines.

To encourage development of the western United States the government granted land to the railroad companies which they could use or sell to assist in the logistics and financing for railroad construction. In 1864 the Northern Pacific Rail Road was approved by Congress and it received a grant of 40 million acres comprised of a swath from 20 to 40 miles wide of every other section of land in a checkerboard pattern. The government retained the other sections for homesteading and other activities. The railroad was free to use what land was necessary and sell or develop the rest. In an effort to raise funds for construction they sold much of the land to immigrant farmers in hopes they would produce products which could then be carried for profit by the railroad. In fact, the railroad forced purchasers of this land to use the rail for transportation of any goods or products produced.

It progressed through fits and starts and bankruptcies for more than 20 years and finally the golden spike was driven by President Grant in western Montana in 1883 thus completing a rail line from coast to coast. In 1888, the first train passed through the just completed Stampede Pass Tunnel connecting Tacoma and Seattle with Minneapolis Saint Paul Minnesota across the northern tier of the United States.

In 1884 coal was discovered in Roslyn lying in narrow seams between the layers of the Teanaway sandstone formation. By 1886 hundreds of immigrants had been attracted for the dangerous job of hard rock mining and supplying coal for the railroad. They were of Italian, German, and Welsh ethnicity. A few years later coal was discovered in Cle Elum and by the turn of the century when the mines were developed by the railroad, large numbers of Croats, Italians, Poles, and Slovaks had arrived to work the mines. By 1910 the Cle Elum population had reached almost 3,000 with great ethnic diversity.

The Northern Pacific Railroad had formed the Northwest Improvement Company in 1897 to handle the non-railroad coal mining and mineral development for the company. In 1900 almost a million acres of railroad land was sold by the cash poor NPR owner Sam Hill to Frederick Weyerhaeuser establishing the western property base of this massive industrial company.

Obviously one of the major needs of this new struggling company was manpower. Trees had to be cut for construction materials and road ties. Tunnels had to be engineered and bored. Coal had to be located, mined, transported to fuel the engines. Fortunately, the timber, gravel, rock, and coal were available on land now owned by the railroad. Most of this work was contracted out to private companies closely supervised by the railroad with much of the labor provided by these immigrants of European ancestry.

So much for the history lesson!

Dominic was a member of the fourth generation of his Croatian family that had come to the Roslyn area in the 1880s. All the male members had been involved with the mines in some capacity. But time marches on and by 1957 the last coal mine in upper Kittitas County had closed. The population had stabilized and most of his family had moved on to other careers such as logging, Forest Service, county jobs and small businesses.

His business and home had been in the Roslyn area known as duck town. The family had been a little dysfunctional and had gradually drifted apart and gone their separate ways. In his retirement, he lived alone in his old house which was built back in the early 1900 mining days. Disaster struck when he had a minor stroke. He quickly recovered fairly well and returned to his usual grumpy self. He was, however, mostly confined to a wheelchair so he had to hire and depend on a patient faithful housekeeper to come in several times a week to clean up and check on him.

His best friend and companion was a big happy black lab cross named Ernie. If Dominic was feeling grumpy and growled at him, Ernie just grinned and wagged his tail and the grumpiness just rolled off like water from a duck's back.

It was difficult for him or the housekeeper to bring Ernie in to the clinic and the family was not much help so I made house calls for any problems or needs that Ernie might have.

Dominic called one day saying that Ernie had been having major accidents in the house usually by the back door. Ernie was a clean well-trained dog so this was certainly out of character and I agreed to drive out and check on the situation.

Ernie gave a "There's someone at the door", kind of bark when I knocked. Dominic wheeled over to let me in. When I looked at Ernie to *size him up,* I was pretty sure I know what the problem was. It has been a long winter and there had been almost no outside time. Ernie was Dominick's best and perhaps only friend and Dominick rewarded his loyalty by giving him unlimited treats. The garbage can in the cluttered kitchen was almost full of empty bags and boxes that had contained all sorts of dog snacks and treats. He had gotten huge. Perhaps 30 lbs. overweight. As a test I, went over and open the back door and he followed me that far. But there was a fairly long and steep flight of stairs out into the backyard. When I encouraged him to descend, he whined and wagged his tail but could only manage the steps when I supported him a little bit by using his strong tail like a steadying suitcase handle.

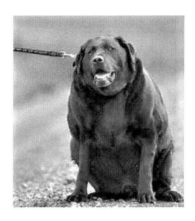

Often a physician or veterinarian gains much valuable medical information by asking questions. I asked Dominic if Ernie had been gaining weight.

He said, "Yes. He is looking a little plump." I asked him what he fed him and he said, "I ain't no animal abuser. I keep his food and water dish full all the time and I give him treats and snacks whenever he begs for them."

There was little question as to what the problem had been. It had been a long cold winter and I'm sure that the steps into the backyard had been snow-covered and icy. Dominic and Ernie had been housebound all winter and the dog had gotten no exercise and also as much food as his stomach could handle.

So how do you retrain an owner? Ernie had been quite successful training Dominic to give into all his requests. But Dominic didn't want to hear me tell him that he was killing his dog with kindness. I said we are going to have to take away at least 1/3 of his caloric intake.

I could see the grumpiness and defiance instantly appear on his face and he said, "I ain't gunna starve my best friend."

I tried to explain that he had gotten so heavy that he was unable and unwilling to navigate the stairs. When the need arose, he headed in the right direction but only got as far as the back door where the accidents were happening with increasing frequency.

I checked on him in 2 weeks but could not identify any improvement. The kitchen was clean and free of empty dog food bags and snack boxes but I noticed there seem to be some new ones in the garbage can on the back porch. I think that Dominic had tried to hide the evidence before I arrived. The housekeeper arrived when I was there and we went off into another part of the house where she and I could have a private conversation beyond Dominic's hearing.

Over the next two weeks she and I both tried to persuade Dominic to ease up on his feeding. I told Dominic, "I know your housekeeper is doing the best that she can but when I come in the front door your house smells like a doggy outhouse. Ernie still can't get up and down the stairs to relieve himself in the backyard. I told him that the extra weight is hard on his heart and his pulse is elevated. He pants all the time because he has an inch of blubber insulation covering his body. He has had some bladder infections because he is trying not to have mistakes and is holding his urine way too long. He is kind of an old man and has some arthritis and this additional weight is making it even more painful for him to get around."

Finally, he grumbled, "Okay, smart guy. You win! Damn it! What do I have to do?"

We were finally starting to get through to him. We devised a plan and Dominic begrudgingly agreed to it.

I jokingly, but never the less with serious intent, said, "If you don't follow through with this plan, I will have you arrested for animal abuse."

He determinedly replied but with a sly grin on his face said, "I'd like to see you try."

We did our best to determine what an ideal weight for Ernie would be. Almost all pet food manufacturers have recommendations on the packaging for how many cups or calories to feed a dog based on the type of breed and its size. Pet food manufacturers don't want the dogs eating their food to look skinny so they tend to be slightly generous on the food recommendations. Inevitably, it comes down to how many calories per day a dog should consume so we set up prepackaged baggies of food and snacks to last for a week. We put the reminder of the snacks and food upstairs where Dominic would not be able to reach them. Thus, he was trapped. If he over fed there would not be enough food to last the week and poor Ernie would have to go without. In reality it wouldn't have harmed him to miss a day or so of food. For each day there were 4 baggies. A morning meal, and evening meal, a morning's worth of snacks, and an afternoon's worth of snacks.

We told Dominic the obvious. "If you give Ernie all the snacks at once, they would soon be gone whereas if you give him one snack every hour the snacks will last all day and hopefully Ernie will feel happier and less abused."

I called once a week to see how things were going and was able to schedule it for the time when the housekeeper was also there so I could talk with her as well. After two hard months for Ernie and Dominic and also too harder months for the housekeeper, because Dominic threatened to fire her because she was making him being mean to his dog, I got the report I was hoping for.

You could hear the joy in Dominic's voice when he said, "This past week Ernie has been making it up and down the porch steps and there have been no accidents in the house."

I congratulated him on his good work and said, "It must be nice to have a clean smelling house again and I know that your dog is in better health.

His reply was, "Yes. it certainly is. Can I take him off this damn diet now Doc?"

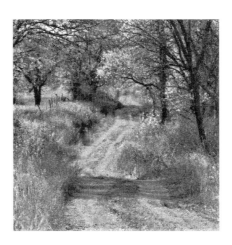

HISTORIC TRAILS AND ROADS OF KITTITAS COUNTY

SIGNIFICANT DATES

1804   President Jefferson sent Meriwether Lewis and William Clark on the Corps of Discovery Expedition to claim territory, establish fur trade, and make scientific discovery.

1814   Fur Trader Alexander Ross entered Kittitas Valley to trade for horses and encountered a massive encampment of perhaps 10,000 Indians near mouth of Naneum Creek.

1853   Washington became a territory.

1855   Treaty of 1855 ceded most of traditional Yakama land in eastern Washington to US government and 14 tribes and bands were confederated into the Yakama Nation. The Confederated Nations were allowed to retain only about 20% of their traditional lands.

1860's   Cattle ranching developed in Kittitas Valley. The most noteworthy cattleman was Ben Snipes.

1863   Ferguson County was created including most of present Yakima and Kittitas counties.

1865   Ferguson County was eliminated and Yakima County created.

1867   Snoqualmie Pass Road was completed.

1867   Frederick Ludi and John Goller were the first non-Indian settlers in the Kittitas Valley building a cabin on the present site of Ellensburg.

1870   AJ Splawn and Ben Burch established Robber's Roost in a small log cabin.

1871   John Shoudy and his wife Mary ELLEN Shoudy (Ellensburg) bought the store and eventually founded Ellensburgh. Note spelling.

1873   Gold was discovered in Swauk Creek.

1883   Coal was discovered in Cle Elum area.

1883   Kittitas County was created.

1887   Northern Pacific Railroad was completed over Stampede Pass.

1889   Washington became a state.

FIRST PEOPLE

Native Americans had lived in the Wenas and Kittitas Valleys for thousands of years. By the 1730's they had acquired horses for transportation from Spanish settlements in the southwest and had a permanent winter settlement at the confluence of Wenas Creek and the Yakima River where they fished. The Wenas Valley had abundant native grasses and was an important feeding area for the Northern Yakama horse herds especially in the winter. They also had long established trail systems that allowed for trade and cultural exchange with Puget Sound and coastal tribes. Snoqualmie Pass was frequently traveled route and Colockum Pass and the Columbia River provided routs for exchanges to the north and east. These routes were also important means for connecting with potential brides and husbands. There was extensive intermarrying between the tribes throughout the whole region.

The first non-Indians traveled through the area in the 1810s and were mostly trappers and fur traders on their way into Hudson Bay territory to the north. Settlers began arriving in numbers during the 1850s. In the Treaty of 1855, Washington Territorial Governor Isaacs Stevens forced the Yakamas, under chief Kamiakin, to cede 11 million acres to the US government and retain only 1.3 million acres for their reservation. They did however retain the right to hunt and fish and their usual and accustomed places.

In Kittitas County there were numerous family settlements of the Kittitas Band of the Yakama Nation. Sites include: Lake Cle Elum, Salmon La Sac, confluence of Yakima and Cle Elum Rivers, Cle Elum, the mouths of Taneum Creek, Manastash Creek, Reecer Creek, Wilson Creek, Naneum Creek, Cariboo Creek, Shushuskin Canyon, mouth of Yakima River, and Badger Pocket. Some were summer camps and some were seasonal for gathering of roots such as camas, biscuit root and balsam root or berries such as black berries and huckleberries.

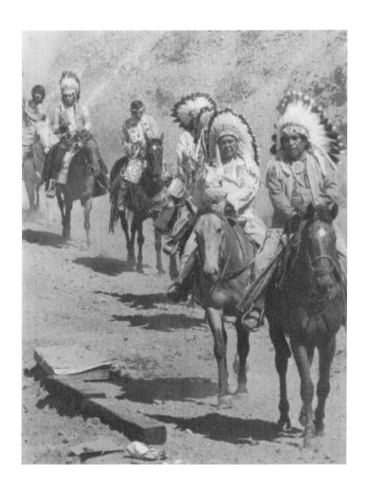

TRAILS

In 1853 David Longmire was a member of the Longmire-Byles party of 36 wagons which were the first to travel over Naches pass. They had to ford the Naches River 68 times. They reached a point where the only way forward was to lower the wagons down over a cliff but they didn't have enough rope. So, they slaughtered some of their oxen and used the hides to extend their rope. David Longmire and his family eventually settled in Yelm and later homesteaded near Longmire Springs by the West entrance to Mt. Rainier National Park and also purchased land in the Wenas Valley.

By the 1840s the Northern Yakamas band led by Chief Owhi (Owhi Gardens in Wenas Valley) had traded for seed and cattle from Fort Steilacoom and Fort Nisqually and were active agriculturists raising corn, barley, potatoes squash and melons and even had irrigation projects (learned from Catholic missionaries) using Wenas Creek water. As the area developed the main occupation for settlers was cattle and sheep ranching but the markets were basically in the Puget Sound area or gold fields of British Columbia, Idaho, and Montana. Using Indian trail systems, cattle were driven over Snoqualmie and Naches Passes to get the cattle to market. To get to Snoqualmie Pass they were driven up the Wenas Valley, up a side canyon to Ellensburg Pass, down the Umptanum Valley into Shushuskin Canyon and then into the Kittitas Valley. From there they were driven up the Yakima River and eventually to Lake Ketchelus. On some occasions they were even forced to swim the length of the lake which was smaller then, not having yet been impounded. From there up and over Snoqualmie Pass, they eventually arrived for market in the Puget Sound area. There was no meat tenderizer.

Cattleman of that era included David Longmire (Longmire entrance to Mt Rainier National Park), A J Splawn (Robbers Roost in early Ellensburg), and Ben Snipes (Snipes Bank in Ellensburg and Roslyn).

ROADS

In the 1850's as the area developed, miners and settlers petitioned for improved roads in the area and in 1853 Congress appropriated $20,000 for a road from Fort Walla Walla to Fort Steilacoom. Secretary of State Jefferson Davis (later to become President of the Confederate States) directed Captain George McClellan (General McClellan of the Battle of Antietam) to survey routes for rail and ground transportation. The route from the Wenas valley up over Umptanum ridge was called the Shushuskin Road after a Yakama Indian who lived at the mouth of Shushuskin Canyon. The first stagecoaches traveled over it in 1873. The grades were fairly easy but it was rather circuitous so in 1882 a Wenas Valley settler name Jacob Durr built a toll road from the lower Wenas Valley up over Umptanum Ridge, down across Umptanum Creek and eventually joining the Shushuskin Road as it drops down into the Kittitas Valley. It was a difficult and expensive undertaking for the time. This route initially crossed the Yakima River at the Manastash Ford (Riverbottom Area) but Durr eventually built a wooden bridge near the present site of the Upper River Bridge (KOA). These routes (Durr and Shushuskin) allowed a stagecoach to travel from The Dalles Oregon 154 miles all the way to Ellensburg. One driver said, "There is no hell in the hereafter; it lies between The Dalles and Ellensburg".

The Durr road was considerably shorter than the Shushuskin Trail route but involved steeper terrain and tight switchbacks. It was necessary to develop turntables (very wide flat spaces at the end of switchbacks which are still evident today) so that the 4 and 6 horse teams required to pull the stagecoach or freight wagons could swing around the corners. Some of the first loads hauled from The Dalles over the Durr Road weighed 1200 lbs. and were to supply goods for sale at Mr. Shoudy's store in Ellensburg. The freighters were Billy Mills and Phil Olmstead (Olmstead State Park). This road was eventually acquired by Kittitas County and became the main route to Yakima.

Meanwhile a group from the west side of the Cascades including Arthur A. Denny (Denny Creek and Denny Way) and a group from the east side of the Cascades including Walter A. Bull

(Bull Road) developed routes that connected over Snoqualmie Pass.

In 1887 the Northern Pacific Railway built the line over Stampede pass and constructed the Stampede Pass tunnel through the Cascades thus completing a more reliable route through the mountains.

The Colockum Pass road started as an Indian trail from the Kittitas Valley connecting north to the Columbia River just downstream from Wenatchee. As early as the 1860's, Ben Snipes trailed stock north to the gold fields on the Fraser River and the Cariboo in British Columbia. By 1883 it had been upgraded to a rough road used by stagecoaches and freighters. In 1892 steamers on the Columbia River connected the road from Rock Island on to Wenatchee but traffic declined because the NP Railroad had been completed. In 1915 the Sunset Highway went from Ellensburg to Vantage where it crossed the Columbia by ferry, then on to Quincy and then back across the Columbia by another ferry. Colockum Pass was carefully considered as a possible better route but it was steep, dangerous, and rugged. Blewett Pass was completed in 1922 and Colockum Pass road reverted to the rough, rocky, and miserable road that it is today.

Washington Territory became a state in 1889 and in 1913 the state legislature allocated funds to open state highways, one of which left Seattle and progressed up the South Fork of the Snoqualmie River and over Snoqualmie Pass to Cle Elum. This was called the Sunset Highway (Sunset Cafe in Cle Elum). In 1922 it eventually continued through Virden (Lauderdale Junction) to the mining area around Liberty and over Old Blewett Pass to Wenatchee, north to Waterville, and east through Davenport to Spokane. The Inland Empire Highway left Virden north of Ellensburg and followed the old Shushuskin Road on to Yakima. It then went through Pasco, Walla Walla and up through Pullman and eastern Washington on to Spokane and the Canadian border. Eventually this section was included in the Yellowstone Trail which had the motto "Plymouth Rock to Puget Sound" and which was conceived in 1912. These named but strangely circuitous routes through Washington served to connect all the major cities with well-built two-lane roadways. My father would have traveled these routes in 1928 when he traveled from Tacoma to Walla Walla to attend Whitman College.

STAGECOACHES

Stagecoaches were usually pulled by four horses and carried 6 to 12 passengers. Two passengers might ride outside on the back and one possibly up-front riding shot gun with the driver. The driver held four reins typically in his left hand (one rein for each horse) and the whip in his right hand. The reins were connected to the outside of the bits while the inside of the bit is connected to the adjacent horse's bit by a short strap. Thus, if a horse on the left was reined to the left, the horse on the right was connected at the bit and had to follow. Coaches were mounted on sleds for winter travel on snowy and icy roads. There were leather curtains over the windows when the weather was cold. They averaged about five miles an hour and could cover 60 to 70 miles in a day. Some stagecoaches had steel springs to cushion the ride while others like the Concorde Stagecoach had leather slings to support the coach which gave more of a swinging ride instead of a jolting ride. Mechanical breaking was provided by a leather covered shoe which pressed against the steel rims of the rear wheels. It was a dirty, miserable, rough, exhausting, sleepless but necessary means of travel. Passengers could be tossed about inside the coach like potatoes in a sack.

A Concorde weighed about a ton and cost between $1500 and $1800. *Swing* or *remount* stations were about 12 miles apart and were locations were fresh teams were swapped in. *Home* stations were about 50 miles apart and were often somebody's home where food and overnight lodging could be provided. Drivers also usually switched at these locations. There is a former swing or remount station about 1 mile east of Ellensburg Pass on Umptanum Road.

Railroad supplanted stagecoaches in many areas but in more remote areas stagecoach travel continued until they were replaced by automobiles in the early 1900s.

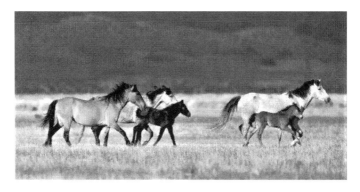

HISTORY OF HORSES IN KITTITAS VALLEY

Known horse ancestry starts with Eohippus, a 30 lb. dog sized grazing animal with 3 toes.

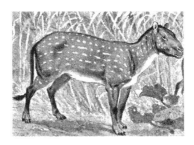

Over a period of 50 million years it evolved into Equus simplicidens, fossilized remains of which were found in Idaho at the Hageman Fossil Beds in 1928. The modern horse developed in North America during the Pleistocene epoch (3.5 – 2.5 million years ago) and it migrated over the Bering land bridge into Asia and Europe. Now, fast forward to the last incursion of the Cordilleran Ice Sheet into North America of 12,000 to 15,000 years ago. Due to changing climate (I doubt that this one was caused by man), and hunting pressure, the modern Equus, like the wooly mammoth, became extinct in North America. However, it had survived and prospered in Asia and more importantly in Europe.

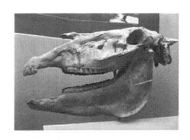

The Europeans apparently had refined and improved horses and when the Silk Road was established in 2nd Century BCE, it was important for trade, but it also allowed horses to be brought from Europe back to Asia. The Chinese needed them to combat the horse mounted Mongolians. The Mongolians had invented the iron stirrup which greatly improved their horsemanship.

By the late 1400's horses had been absent from the Americas for 12,000 to 15,000 years. Christopher Columbus appeared and made four exploratory voyages to the Caribbean. On the second voyage he brought 25 horses from Spain to Cuba and Hispaniola (Haiti and Dominican Republic) and thus reintroduced the horse to the Western Hemisphere where they had initially evolved. (He also brought smallpox for which the **Indians** traded back tobacco and syphilis). The first horse breeding colony was established in Cuba. One reference with genetic documentation says these horses were of Sorraia and Galicia breeding named after those regions of Spain. Later explorers brought more horses and in 1519 Cortez established a breeding colony on the island of Hispaniola which he used as a base of operations to explore and plunder Mexico.

The remnants of these horses (16 brought by Cortez) became the Galiceno breed. They were not selectively bred but rather bred freely more along the lines of survival of the fittest. They are short (12 – 13.5 hands), small (600 – 750 lbs.), short backed, narrow but deep chested, usually solid colored or roan, and may have a dorsal stripe, shoulder cross, and zebra striped legs. Blood lines have been found to be surprisingly pure with little evidence of interbreeding. The Spanish Colonial Horse was said to be clannish staying together as a herd and avoiding mixing with other horses. They were used for transportation, dray, pack, and in the mines by the colonial explorers and settlers. By the 1600's as these horses were released, stolen, or escaped they developed into the Spanish Mustang including the Kiger of Oregon, the Sulfur of SW Utah, and the Pryor Mountain of Montana.

In 1539 De Soto brought horses to Florida which developed into the Florida Cracker Horse so named for the *crack* of the bullwhip wielded by its rider while herding cattle. Spanish rancheros had thousands of horses and the Spanish government established laws forbidding horse ownership by Indians. However, the Apache and Navaho had acquired horses and were excellent horsemen by the mid 1600's. They traded with the plains Comanche who, realizing the animal's value, became adept at raiding Mexican rancheros. The horses were free ranging, easily rounded up, and may have been stolen at the rate of 30,000 per year.

Within 50 years the horse had spread north to the Shoshone, Crow, Flatheads and Nez Perce. Native American culture made a quantum leap in a few short years from a seasonal tribal foot migration to horse based. By 1730, in our region the Nez Perce had become proficient horsemen. By 1760, horses could be found as far north as the Calgary region of western Canada.

In 1814 a fur trader named Alexander Ross rode over Manastash Ridge into the valley to trade for horses and stumbled upon an enormous gathering of Indians. They may have numbered 10,000 and were encamped over a 6-mile area from the mouth of Naneum Canyon to Cariboo Creek. There may have been 3 horses for every Indian. Our valley was one of the few places where camas bulbs, kouse (known as biscuitroot or Lomatium), and bitter root could be found in harvestable quantities. Arrowleaf Balsamroot, (we see its yellow sunflower like bloom in the local foothills in early spring), was also harvested for its oil rich seeds and starchy tap root. Tribes from the Great Plains, coastal Washington, British Columbia interior, Nez Perce, and the many sub tribes of the Yakamas were all present for trading, socializing, horse racing, games, food gathering, councils, dancing, singing, and perhaps for mate finding. Apparently if you know where to look, there are still signs of their horse racing track.

In 1859 James Kinney came to an area in Yakima and Benton counties between the Yakima and Columbia Rivers and observed the knee-high lush grass waving in the breeze and the large herds of wild horses and said, "This surely is a horse heaven." Thus, the name, the Horse Heaven Hills. The Kittitas valley eventually turned to fenced pastures and hay production and the Horse Heavens, Palouse and Columbia Basin turned to wind farms, grain, fruit, and grapes.

The Spanish mustang line has been greatly diluted by other breeds turned loose or escaped and all are in peril of suffering and starvation. They have exceeded the carrying capacity of their grazing ranges because of overpopulation or drought. There is no one solution pleasing to all concerned individuals but the present situation is untenable. It has been said that the Yakima Nation Reservation has a horse carrying capacity of 1500 horses and there may be as many as 10,000.

Locally, cattle were part of the backbone of the economy and you can't handle cattle without horses. Much of the valley was partitioned into large self-sufficient cattle operations and each had its own herd of working and breeding stock. Early horses in the valley probably had some draft blood in them and may have partial origin in pioneer wagon pulling stock. Mix in some native Spanish descendent horse blood, quarter horse and a little thoroughbred and you have the beginnings of the breed that helped *Win the West*.

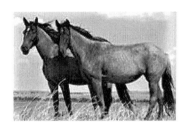

European immigrants brought horses to America. The first were small, due to the limited space on sailing vessels. As commerce and transportation needs arose larger draft breeds were imported in large numbers. Quarter Horses date back to the mid 1600's when native horses of Spanish origin were crossed with English breeds of Thoroughbred type. Their quickness, agility, good natured disposition and cow sense were a perfect fit for the historic cattlemen of our valley. The zenith of horses in the Kittitas valley might be said to culminate with the Ellensburg Rodeo

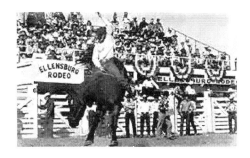

Some of the first rodeos were casual events after annual cattle roundups. Cattle ranged freely and herds often mixed together so they were gathered for branding and sorting. Boys being boys, this was an opportunity to exhibit their skills in riding, roping and bulldogging. On June 14, 1923 local farmers, businessmen, ranchers, and Yakima Indians 500 strong with 200 horses turned out for a *field day* to construct the Ellensburg Rodeo Arena.

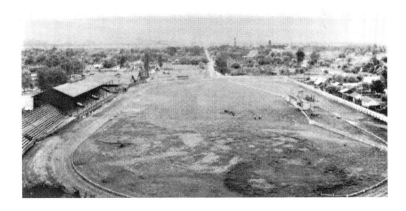

Local pioneer names for buildings, businesses, roads, and canyons are still evident and all were associated with horses.

Elizabeth and James Ferguson came to the Kittitas Valley in 1867 and established a ranch on Naneum Creek on what is now called Ferguson Road. Their boys made a living gathering wild horses and herding cattle in the region. Ben Ferguson and his brother staged impromptu Sunday rodeos in the 1920's about four miles east of town near Ferguson Road which led to community involvement and building the rodeo grounds.

Cifford Kaynor, newspaperman, was the owner/editor of The Evening Record which became the Ellensburg Daily Record. He was a strong promotor of the Ellensburg Rodeo and the High Line Canal irrigation project.

Phillip Fitterer arrived via the Oregon Trail and married Emma Daverin, who, with her twin brother, may have been the first white children born in the Kittitas Valley. Phillip and his brother Frank managed the Horton Hotel which was lost during the great fire of 1889. The process of rebuilding connected them with furniture retailers and thus the establishment of Fitterer Brothers Furniture Store in 1896 which had a stable of horses for furniture delivery.

The Nason and SoHappy families have ancestral connections to the Kittitas Valley and celebrate their Meeting Ground tradition with dancing and horse racing activities during the Ellensburg Rodeo.

Veterinarian Dr. H. F. Pfenning was the first superintendent.

Local cowboys Howard Thomas and Frank Woods were early participants.

Horses continue to be part of the fabric of the Kittitas Valley only now they do pleasure trail riding, three day eventing or horse trials, western dressage, competitive trail riding, endurance rides, ranch horse competitions 4-H shows, games, drill teams and are a major contributor to the local economy. Local cowboys and cowgirls achieve national prominence in their specialty rodeo events such as roping and barrels. It should be noted that a new truck and horse trailer can cost almost as much as a small house.

Where would we be without horses?

DVM (Retired) Writer

509-899-1145

newschwander@gmail.com

NATURE VS NURTURE

act a mother has on her offspring has been well
new knowledge continues to be unraveled. There is a
about how rat mothers take care of their pups. In
of rats, it is noted that the mothers take good care of
id spend more time grooming, nursing, and especially
igine being licked by a rat!) Other mothers spend less
:r pups and grooming is rather perfunctory. It seemed
able trait because good mothers raise daughters who
y became good mothers while the opposite was true
of the poor mothers.

In a recent study pups were grafted from a poor mother soon
after birth onto a good mother who did the usual good job of
grooming the adopted pups. Conveniently, lab rats reach sexual
maturity between 5 and 8 weeks and have a gestation period of
three weeks so it doesn't take long to determine whether traits are
heritable. The results in this study were startling. The rats from
the poor mothers which were grafted onto good mothers and
therefore received good care, proved to be good mothers when
they eventually reached sexual maturity and delivered pups. Had
they been left with their poor mothers they also would have
proven to be poor mothers. Inversely, if you took rat pups from a
good mother and grafted them onto a poor mother, they would
develop the characteristics of their adoptive mother and her poor
mothering skills.

These studies elucidate what's called the plasticity of the
genome. Historically, we would have thought that traits were firm
and depended on the genetic makeup of the DNA. We are now
learning that in many circumstances a genome may display
different traits based on early maternal interaction. This is called

epigenetics. An analogy might be that we are dealt a hand of DNA cards but stress to the mother during pregnancy or to the newborn releases or contributes chemicals that can change the DNA queen of spades into the queen of hearts.

Now look at the situation from a species and individual rat survival point of view. The poor mother is more likely to be thinner, more nervous, and vigilant and thus more likely to survive harsh or adverse circumstances in a dangerous world. If a pup from a good mother is grafted onto the poor mother that pup will have modifications in the expression of its genome that will better enable it to survive under more hazardous conditions. Conversely, rats raised in a stress-free laboratory environment by good mothers have a poor chance of surviving in the wild.

I am quite sure a similar thing happens with kittens. In a hypothetical situation, you observe a young obviously pregnant female cat disappear into your woodpile during a winter snow storm. A few days later you see the no longer pregnant cat depart never to return. You disassemble the woodpile and find 5 cold scrawny little kittens struggling to survive. You bring them in and feed them and keep them warm but to your disappointment as they mature you find they are timid, fearful, and unlikely to become a pleasing friendly pet. In other words, they will be just like their mother. If you were able to find another cat or even a dog who would accept them and nurture them and lick them you would find that some of these kittens mature with the sweet personality of their adopted mother. Maybe the human surrogate mothers should learn to lick the kittens. Some hairball medicine might be advisable.

The explanation for this involves the study of epigenetics. Genes may sometimes be in an active or inactive state. Chemicals or external stressors can cause them to transition from one state to another. Hair color, skin tone, and sociability are all characteristics that can be influenced by this process.

I have a small pretty female cat who resides in my barn and keeps it free of unwanted rodent alien invaders. Her name is DC which is short for Doc's Cat. She was abandoned at a very young age and then rescued from underneath an old abandoned house. She was the prettiest and therefore got the most attention from her rescuer. Her littermates were all neutered but received minimal attention and have proven to be minimally sociable or trusting of human beings. DC in contrast however, enjoys being petted and groomed but resists being picked up and held. As long as she has her feet on something solid where she feels like she is in control she can be loving and attentive. But once you to pick her up, her instinct is to escape. I would say that her epigenetic genome has been partially modified so she is somewhere between a feral cat and a delightfully domesticated house cat. She will come into my house and explore a little bit but soon wants to be back outside into her comfort zone. Her early childhood (kittenhood) development partially reprogramed the expression of her DNA.

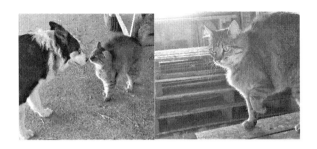

Most Cattlemen, at some time or another, have had a least favorite cow. These are dangerous animals under any circumstances and are just as likely to charge you as they are to avoid you. Add their calf to the mix and they can be especially testy. Statistically their calves will display the same unfriendly characteristics. If it is a bull calf it will be castrated in the fall and eventually move on to take up residence at Wendy's or McDonalds. If it is a heifer it will likely be retained as a replacement heifer and now you can have 2nd and 3rd generation cows that can be difficult to deal with.

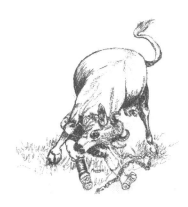

Typically, animals receive numbered ear tags at birth to help identify them. One rancher had cows with numbers 27, 127, and 227. I remember him saying, "Watch out for 227. She's just as nasty as her mother and grandmother. I think I would sooner tangle with a nest of ground hornets."

One year the granddaughter rejected her newborn calf for unknown reasons. Ranchers sometimes keep a gentle old Holstein cow around to use as a wet nurse. Under her calming attentive mothering this calf developed a personality more like that of her stepmother.

There may be another related analogy from nature. It is a well-known fact that cattle somehow seem to sense the onset of a major storm. I suspect it relates to the dramatic change in atmospheric pressure. Cattle that are close to term in their pregnancy often deliver their calves just before the onset of the storm. If things don't improve and the weather is severe enough it is not uncommon for them to abandon their calves. One explanation of the situation is that nature sacrifices the newborn so that the reproductively mature animal can survive to produce again the next year. Now consider the animal, typically a heifer having her first calf, who refuses to care for her newborn calf. It seems likely that the stress has activated the pituitary adrenal axis which kicked in with the resulting high cortisol levels causing her aberrant behavior.

Consider a human infant born to poverty, a single parent, or an environment of drugs and violence. The deck is dramatically stacked against them. A study by a Stanford pediatrician showed striking increases in the rate of autism, ADHD, asthma, diabetes, heart disease, cancer, depression, suicide, decreased life expectancy in a child born to a mother enduring high stress during her pregnancy. When some of these children were assisted through an intervention by nurturing specialists, it appeared possible to alter or even reverse the impact of their stressful perinatal period.

Who says you can't learn anything from a rat?

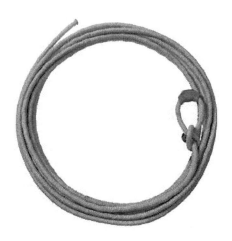

BIG LOOP RODEO

You could see them coming from miles away. At first it was impossible to tell what it was but there was a huge cloud of gray dust like an African haboob inexorably headed our way. We climbed up on a small rise to get a better view and gradually moving shapes began to appear only to disappeared momentarily when they dropped down into a dip in the rugged terrain. When they reappeared, it became obvious that it was a herd of wild horses. You could see their heads, necks, and shoulders lunging up and down as they galloped towards us. Finally, you could recognize their ears. The ears on the horses are for listening and for communicating with their herd mates. The ears on the horses in front were pointed forward in an alert fashion as they scanned the terrain before them. The horses in the middle of the herd had their ears in an intermediate position part way forward and back or one forward and one back as they listened and communicated with horses in front and behind them. They had to avoid the bodies and feet in front of them and find footing for themselves as they galloped. The horses in the swirling cloud of dust bringing up the rear had their ears flat back against their head. Were they watching and listening behind for anything potentially dangerous that might be following them?

However, they weren't really wild horses but rather were owned by local ranchers. They were 1, 2, and 3-year old animals turned out into a huge range area to be given supplemental feed if necessary but mainly to survive and mature on their own. Periodically they would be rounded up to be culled and sold, castrated if appropriate, or retained for training.

If you pick up Highway I 82 South it will take you up and over Manastash Ridge, Umptanum Ridge, and Yakima Ridge through the sage and grassland steppes of Eastern Washington. It passes by Yakima, through the cut in Rattlesnake Ridge at Union Gap, past Tri-Cities and then across the Columbia River at Hermiston. Then you head East on I-84 through Pendleton, up over the Pondarosa pinelands of the Blue Mountains and finally on to Ontario Oregon. Now you pick up Idaho 95 South until you find yourself at Jordan Valley.

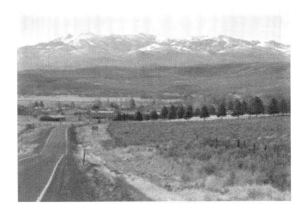

You been driving 7 hours and have covered 425 miles. So, where are you? It has a population of 175 people so you can see why it's called The Empty Corner of Eastern Oregon. They say the phone book has five pages and the library still uses the Dewey Decimal System and has a card catalog. There is a gas station, a shop, a general store, a restaurant, a hotel, courthouse and a school. What more do you need? This is cattle ranch country, horse country, and old-style rodeo country. Modern-day cattle rustling has on occasion transpired here. Cattle can just disappear off into the emptiness. When the terrain is too rough for wheeled vehicles and cattle are spread out over thousands of square miles of grass range, old school cowboy skills are still a valuable commodity. The Big Loop Jordan Valley Rodeo is the local cowboy's opportunity to showcase their skills.

Why is it called the Big Loop Rodeo? Under natural or rodeo circumstances cows and calves tend to run in a straight line and having a fairly short neck and limited agility are not able to dodge a loop thrown at their head. A horse, on the other hand is more agile and probably has better peripheral vision and with its long neck can evade a thrown loop. Consequently, if you are roping range bred horses you have to throw a giant loop in order to catch the horse. One of the tricks to successful roping is too quickly draw the slack to tighten the lariat around the animal's neck. It takes tremendous strength on the part of the cowboy to gather up the slack in this especially long lariat.

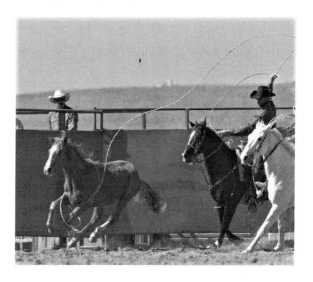

Working horses or cattle out on the range is not a timed event where animals come out of gates or alleyways. In an attempt to imitate more natural conditions, this rodeo gives the cows, horses, or calves an extra-long head start. This means the animals coming out for the contestant have more time to gain speed and attempt escape. Thus, the arena is considerably larger since it was built for the cowboy and not for the rodeo audience. Competitors have to be especially careful when the animal approaches the far end of the arena at high speed that is not crowded because in its attempt to escape it could inadvertently crash into the distant fence. Should this happen the cowboy is immediately disqualified.

Every attempt is made to protect the rodeo stock from injury by overly competitive and aggressive cowboys.

Modern rodeos are exhibitions of the competitor's and the animal's skills and athleticism in front of an audience. I don't believe that there were stopwatches, judges, TV cameras, and announcers during the Golden Age of the western cowboy (after the Civil War and into the later 1800s). The big loop Rodeo attempts to resurrect the atmosphere and techniques of the original cowboys. Initially they were employed to gather and bring the wild cattle from the grasslands of Texas north to be put on the railroad to be shipped east. There was no need to ride bulls. The bulls had a job to do and you tried to stay out of their way. Calves needed to be worked on and you had to catch them wherever you found them. There weren't alleyways keeping them all lined up and ready to run in a straight line. There was a great need for horses but not necessarily a lot of time to train them so the more humane techniques of the modern era did not come into play. Horses were broken because it was the quickest way to turn them into a useful commodity. A cowboy got on a horse and tried to stay on board until the horse quit and accepted the mastery of the rider. There was no need to show off and wave your hands in the air like on a carnival roller coaster ride. Cowboys got on board as best they could and hung onto the saddle horn to prevent getting thrown and to stay on board until the horse gave in. I don't know how they scored the bucking horse rides at the Big Loop Rodeo but the cowboys who hung onto the saddle horn scored just as well or even better than the cowboys who rode in the modern style waving a free arm in the air to help maintain their balance.

The Big Loop Rodeo is held every spring on the third weekend in May. For that rodeo weekend the town is overrun. There is not adequate lodging space within almost a hundred miles so people come with campers, tents, and trailers and park anywhere there is room, even along the shoulders of the highway. They open the school grounds and parking lots to provide additional space for visitors. There is an exorbitant fee of $10 to enter the rodeo grounds and watch. This provides you with the vicarious opportunity to partake in the work and lifestyle of a true western cowboy. On Monday the locals say, "Only 362 days until we do it all over again."

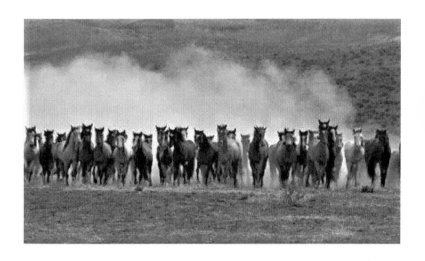

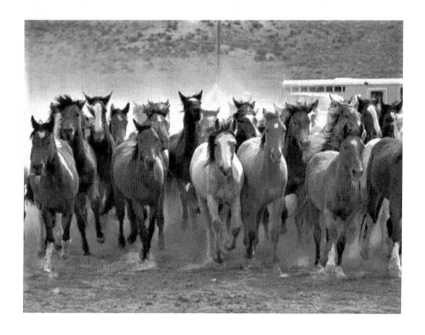

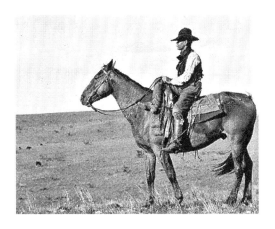

LAST OF THE KIND

They don't build them that way anymore. They lost the blueprint and threw away the mold and all we have left are the stories and memories and some dusty dried-out cracked leather tack in a barn somewhere. There might also be a 1950's vintage white Ford 1-ton stock truck out behind the barn disappearing into the grass and brush with a quail's nest under the hood.

He might have admitted that life could be sometimes hard but he also would have added, "I wouldn't have wanted it any other way." He had everything he needed. First and foremost was a dedicated wife willing to work right alongside him if the need arose. Second was a cow dog versatile enough to work sheep, cows, and horses and who could understand the quiet words, body language, and hand signals of his owner. Third was a horse. It didn't have to be fancy or fast. It had to be steady, dependable, and willing to put in long days either pushing cattle or standing patiently ground tied when his rider did not need him. Fourth was a one-ton horse truck. His wife rode shotgun or was the driver if the truck needed to be ferried to another location. The dog rode up in the horse hay manger if the weather was not too cold. In bad weather it jumped up into the tack space beneath the manger and circled around and around on top of the horse blankets before flopping down and tucking his nose under his tail. And where did the horse go? Why in the horse compartment of course? There was a loading ramp but usually the boss just backed the truck into a ditch and the horse jumped on board.

The rest of the equipment was variable and optional but might include boots, spurs, Wranglers, chap's, a belt with a tarnished silver buckle, snap button shirt, quilted jacket, duster with a wool liner, bandana, leather gloves, lariats, and a battered western felt hat with a thoroughly sweat-stained hatband.

Where did this story begin? Leroy was one of 9 survivors out of 13 births. His parents had homesteaded in 1903 and struggled to survive in the Devils Tower grassland region of eastern Wyoming. They had a few horses for riding and pulling wagons and equipment plus a few beef and dairy cows. Their main source of income, however, was hogs. In those days you couldn't just go down do your local co-op and by bags of starter pig feed. When times were tough and money was short, which was often the case, the pigs came first. The sows and boars had to get out and hustle to forage for whatever they could find to eat. Any extra milk, of course went to the pigs as did anything left over from the kitchen. If times were really tough the family of 15 only ate one meal a day primarily of beans with a little pork fat and crisped skin thrown in for flavor. There was no shortage of lard for anything fried.

There was no power, no water, and no internal combustion engine. No radio, no TV, and no cell phones. People had to talk to each other.

When it came time to market the pigs, since they had no truck for transportation, they had to drive them 40 miles to the nearest railroad at Sundance (yes, of Sundance Kid fame), by horseback assisted by the dogs. Fortunately, pigs are herd animals and don't like to be left behind so they could be slowly moved along stopping frequently for snacking on any available forage. They did it in the winter often over snow because it was easier on the pigs. It only took 3 1/2 days. A horse drawn sled carried hog feed and a place to ride for any pigs that played out. Nobody told them it was going to be a one-way trip.

In a family that large, the children kind of had to raise themselves. You probably teamed up with a sibling closest to you in age. The father was apparently rather abusive and if the kids didn't meet his expectations, he was more than willing to handout corporal punishment. If they were in trouble, they were sent out to cut their own willow switches which he would apply liberally to their backsides.

The family tells one very grim story. It was Leroy's responsibility to bring the milk cows in at evening for milking and his brother's to take them back out to pasture in the morning after milking. One morning about two hours late his brother's horse came in but without a rider. A search located where the horse had fallen but neither his brother or his body was ever found.

Leroy went to school as far as the 8th grade but when he turned 18 there were so many mouths to feed, he was essentially kicked out of the house to make his own way in the world.

The Devils Tower is a basaltic geological formation which was injected up through the underlying sandstone sedimentary layers only about 50 - 60 million years ago. It was made into a national monument in 1909 by Teddy Roosevelt but work was not done to develop it until the 1940's. One of the Leroy's first jobs after escaping the hardship of home life was to work developing hiking trail networks around the monument and through the park.

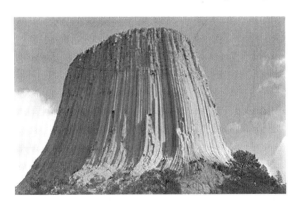

Leroy drifted east through Iowa and on to Illinois where he fell in love with and married his lifetime companion, a city girl. I doubt he ever felt at home in this urban environment as a bus mechanic but there was a wife and growing family to feed. Then one day in a western cattlemen's magazine he spotted an ad for someone looking for ranch help in Washington State. They talked it over and decided to accept the offer for work and packed up for the 1200-mile drive out west.

Leroy's wife, they called her Tiny because she was, said, "The first time I realized I had married a cowboy it was when we loaded the car and Leroy put on his 10-gallon cowboy hat and boots for the drive out west."

The job proved to be a perfect fit. He knew how to handle dogs, horses, cattle, and sheep and could work independently accomplishing any of the myriad livestock related tasks on a large integrated ranch operation.

Now we see the strength, determination, and durability of the man start to manifest itself. On one occasion when chasing cattle out on the range Leroy's horse fell and he wound up under it with a with a broken tibia. It wasn't a terribly serious fracture but, in those days, they put you in a plaster cast to stabilize things until they healed. But after a few days of sitting around doing nothing Leroy couldn't take it anymore and there was work to be done so he filled up the bathtub with water and got in and soaked until he was able to rip the plaster cast off. That afternoon he was back in the saddle out helping move cattle.

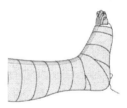

Another story involves a confrontation with an unfriendly cow. Usually cows move away from a horse and would not challenge one. This cow apparently did not read the cow owner's manual and when roped decided to charge the horse. The horse deftly stepped out of the way but the cow was attached to the end of the lariat and circled around entangling the horse, rider, and cow in one big lassoed knot. They all collapsed in a tangled pile with the dog barking at the periphery. All survived the encounter and the cow got shipped that fall out of respect for her personality traits.

Later in life, his heart was causing him some issues and he had to go in for bypass heart surgery. First, they open your chest by splitting your sternum down the middle of your chest. When they are done tuning up the heart, they put you back together again by lacing your split sternum back together with stainless steel wire.

Again, there was work asking to be done and about 10 days later Leroy, with only some Ace bandages around his chest to support it, was back out working cows again.

One of the most indispensable assistants for a cattleman is his dog. Somehow Leroy had a knack for looking at young dogs and picking the one he could communicate with and train to do what was required. It takes a truly remarkable working dog to handle both sheep and cattle. Cattle are tough and it takes a tough dog to occasionally bite their back feet to move and control them. Sheep however are very fragile and physical contact can possibly lead to injury so herding is done by eye contact where the dog positions itself and using body language controls the sheep. I sometimes felt that Leroy and his dog worked so well together that if Leroy wanted the dog to momentarily stop herding and stay where it was, the dog could almost be stopped in the air mid-flight and hover there like a giant black and white humming bird until given another command.

Late in life Leroy finally had to give up his hard-working ways. He got pitched off a horse and landed on his elbow and shoulder. His elbow, humerus, and shoulder were badly damaged. After surgical repair and healing, so much of the range of motion was lost and he was unable to throw a rope anymore.

Once when asked about his hard years of cowboying he said, "It was recreation to me. Fooling with my horses, training my dog, working the cattle, that ain't work. That's just what I do!"

He seemed a little bewildered after he lost his wife, Tiny, in the early 2000s. Three years later at the age of 91, Leroy was gone too. I suspect if you let your imagination wander and watch and listen carefully enough, you can sense that Leroy is out there horseback somewhere working cows and whistling quietly while giving hand signals to his trusty Border Collie companion.

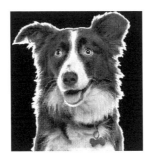

GRUMPY OLD MEN

There is a phrase from the 16th century describing a dog's existence. They would guard homes, were fed scraps and plate scrapings, slept outside, and had short hard lives. Life wasn't much fun. It was *A Dog's Life*. Now, dogs rarely guard homes because they travel first class with their owners. They are fed special foods, sleep on soft quilted cushions, and have long easy lives. The phrase *It's a Dog's Life* has to come to a mean almost the opposite of its old antiquated usage.

I suspect there is a parallel between the dog and the horse regarding the nature of their existence. I think it's fair to say that the modern horse has a pretty easy time of it compared to the *good old days* but life still has its ups and downs. Such was surely the case with Gazon.

He began his life as a 60 lb. long slippery package consisting mainly of legs and ears. His slightly dished nose identified him as an Arabian horse. He wobbled around on his still soft rubbery hooves instinctively knowing that somewhere there was something that would provide nourishment for his stomach if he could only find it and suck on it.

Someone asked, "I wonder what color he is going to be?"

He could only be described as having a light foal hair coat. Was he going to be black? Would it a dark gray? Dapples? Only time would tell.

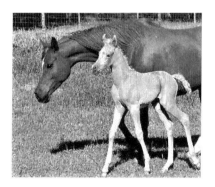

He was soon pronging around the pasture like a gazelle with his tail straight up in the air. When he got hungry, he would maneuver in front of his mother forcing her to stop thus giving him access to the mobile milk dispenser. Life was a busy fascinating time. There were butterflies to smell and chase when they flew off. There were the other foals in the nursery pasture so there was always someone up for a romp. Cottontail rabbits were unwitting playmates as they hopped around nibbling on the choicest bits of clover. There was always something somewhere else the needed closer examination and the only time to do it was right now. Sleeping, eating, learning how to buck and kick and gallop in circles was a full-time occupation.

A year quickly passed but, in that time, he learned halter manners, to enjoy being brushed, and to stand quietly while his hooves were trimmed. When he shed out his winter coat that spring, it became evident that he was going to be very light, almost white gray horse will a slight amount of dappling.

That fall when he was a year-and-a-half-old and fly season was over, he had an appointment with his personal veterinary surgeon for an attitude adjustment. His daddy was still young and didn't require any help entertaining all the mares on the farm. After he got poked with a needle in the neck, he felt strangely wobbly and didn't even feel it when he collapsed in a heap on the ground. He had no idea how long he had been asleep but when he struggled to his feet, he felt surprisingly hungry and soon found some sweet clover to chew on. He was pretty sore *back there* and he felt that something seemed to be missing, but after a few days he forgot all about it.

But he sure loved all the attention he was getting. His mistress would call him in from the pasture, give him a little grain, and give him a good brushing. Then they went into the big covered arena with the nice soft dirt floor for play time and he got to walk, trot, and gallop around in circles. He preferred prancing with his tail and ears up but his mistress discouraged having that much fun. That winter he learned how to wear a saddle and even got to carry his mistress for brief easy workouts in the arena.

The next few years had some ups and downs. There were some long boring periods of training sessions in indoor or outdoor arenas as he learned how to be balanced when carrying a rider, how to respond to rein and leg cues, and comprehend the basic elements of dressage. All the hard work seemed worth it when he had advanced enough to start going to novice horse shows. There were people and horses everywhere. Things were happening and he wanted to be part of it. It made his heart beat faster.

By the time he was seven, his bones had matured and reached their full strength and it was time to start jumping and participating in three day eventing. This involved dressage in an arena, cross country jumping courses, and stadium jumping. It was like any human high-level athletic endeavor and has its roots in comprehensive military cavalry training. Long hours of training and practice paid off when he got to compete against all the other horses. Gazon wasn't a champion but did well enough to keep his owner interested and challenged.

This is when Mother Nature threw Gazon his first major curveball. In spite of being a gelding he still had an overly keen interest in the ladies. One spring he flirted too aggressively with a cranky old mare and she responded by kicking out with both hind feet. One shod hind foot caught him full in the face and that afternoon his veterinarian had to remove his destroyed eye. When he healed it became evident that his high-level jumping days were over because he needed two eyes to accurately measure distances.

Without intending to be mean or catty, people sometimes said, "We'll just put on an eyepatch and he can be in Arabian pirate horse."

However, he was now middle-aged and was just one horse in a large stable. His services were no longer required.

The next hand of cards he was dealt had a queen of hearts in it. She and her two daughters lived in the neighborhood near the stable. When they visited the stable one day, Gazon's owner explained what had happened, and said "I don't know what we're going to do with him."

The lady with the two little girls said hopefully, "I am a divorced single parent and money is pretty tight but maybe we could buy him with time payments."

Gazon's owner said, "That would be perfect. How does $1 a month for a year sound? There is not much market for a one-eyed pirate Arabian jumper and I can't imagine a better situation for him than to go home with you and your daughters."

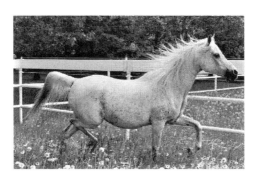

And so, the fourth happy stage in his life began. He was well cared for and loved and still got to go to lower-level shows where he got to gracefully gallop around arenas and jump over some easy small jumps carrying his new young mistress. Little girls, however, grow up and discover boys and mothers get busy providing, so Gazon's show days came to an end. However, another learning opportunity presented itself because the girl's mother and her new husband liked trail riding. Mountain trails along streams, up ridges, and through grassy meadows are certainly more interesting then arenas but it was a challenge to be on the lookout for any danger if you only had one eye. That's when being part of a herd became especially important. Three eyes are *almost* as good as four.

He probably told his fellow herd members, "If you will watch out for me when we're on the trail, I'll be more than glad to pay you back by grooming and nibbling on your neck when we get back to our home pasture."

He loved trail riding but his age and the stress on his joints from show jumping were becoming evident. Osteoarthritis had begun to develop in his left hock. He could still travel rather comfortably but if he came to a log in the trail, he could get his front legs over but was not able to bend the hind leg enough to get it to clear the obstacle. On one occasion he got high centered over a log with his front legs on one side and his hind legs on the other. The riders did not want to cut the ride short almost before it began and there was no way around the log so they decided to see if they could help him out of this predicament. With her tugging rhythmically on the halter and getting Gazon to sway forward and back while he put his shoulder underneath the horse's butt from behind, they were able to boost his hindquarters up and over the log. I am sure all the chipmunks and squirrels watching from the sidelines made small chirps and squeaks of applause that the team had overcome the obstacle.

Even this pleasant phase of his life eventually had to come to an end. He seemed comfortable out grazing in the pasture and could even come slowly trotting for his share of grain but even his trail riding days were obviously over. If he did too much one day, the next day would prove to be very uncomfortable for him.

A fortuitous series of events opened the next chapter of his life. George and Harriet had retired to a small rural acreage at the mouth of the Teanaway River Valley. George was exceedingly grumpy and could be very disagreeable but Harriet more than made up for it with her polite cheerfulness. They had two old retired horses to keep them company and give them something to do. In spite of being a curmudgeon, George truly loved his horses and took excellent care of them. It gave him a reason to get up and be alive every morning. Buck was a large draft cross buckskin and Pony was a small 300-pound pony. It was pretty hard to keep their names straight. They were inseparable and were the Danny and Arnold of the equine world.

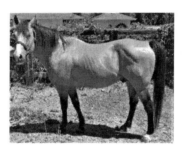 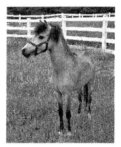

One morning Pony did not wake up and come out of his stall. He was found curled up in permanent sleep in the deep soft straw alongside his manger. Danny stood nearby as if guarding his friend.

George and Harriet called up explaining what had happened and said, "We can't get Buck to even come out of his stall in the barn. He's drinking but eating very little. If we can't get him going, he'll just starve himself to death. Do know anyone might need a retirement home for a horse?"

I said, "I just happen to know someone really well who might need a retirement situation for a horse. That someone is me. Let me talk it over with my ladies but I'll bet we can bring Gazon out this Saturday afternoon."

We delivered our old friend that Saturday. I didn't really know what to expect. We unloaded him and let him graze a little bit on the edge of the driveway. We led him up to the Dutch type stall door to let the old-timers get acquainted. They sniffed noses and snorted and then all hell broke loose. They squealed and screamed and struck out making a us fear they were going to tear the door right off its hinges.

George, with his typical sarcasm, said, "That certainly went well!"

Hoping that time and safe but separate proximity might help, we decided to lock the two old boys side by side in stalls in the barn with a high secure wall between them. They would be able to see and smell each other but not harm themselves or hopefully the wall.

I said, "Let's cross our fingers and give them a week and see if they can learn to play well with others."

Harriet called midweek and said, "Well, the barn is still standing. It was pretty noisy with squeals and thumps for the first two days but things have quieted down now and they both seemed glad to see us when we visit them in the morning for grain in their solitary confinement."

I said, "That's certainly good news. I'll come out Saturday afternoon and we'll give them another chance."

Saturday dawned warm, sunny, with just a slight breeze keeping the air moving. It was a perfect day for a saunter out to the meadow for a mid-afternoon snack of clover and grass. We opened the barn doors and but had to step back to get out of the way. Both horses bolted out and at first, they were so excited just to be out the barn and on the grass that they ate nonstop for 10 minutes. It seems like they almost didn't stop to breathe and had their vegetable conveyor belt running from their lips directly to their stomach. Finally, having satisfied those initial desires, they stopped for a moment and looked up and seemed almost startled to see each other. They walked quickly towards each other and we feared for another equine confrontation. They stopped a short distance from each other sniffed and snorted each other's breath, squealed and postured but didn't strike out. Slowly, cautiously they sidled up alongside each other until they stood head to tail and then began nibbling each other's backs at the withers just where the mane stops. I call this nagging. Gazon, having satisfied his social needs, put his head and began grazing but Buck wasn't done and began licking his new pasture mate. We stood there becoming more and more amused as we watched the scene before us. Over the next half hour, it appeared that Buck had almost licked every square inch of Gazon's white body.

I said, "I thought Gazon was pretty clean and white having spent the time in the barn but I guess Buck decided he needed a bath."

Harriet said, "It's just like a mother with a small child with a dirty spot on the child's face. The mother looks around to make sure nobody is watching and then gives the child's face a quick spit bath. I guess Buck just gave Gazon one giant spit bath."

We all went in and sat on the deck behind George and Harriet's house. We could look out over the pasture and observe the two new best friends. Harriet had luckily timed things perfectly and went into the kitchen to take two homemade loaves of bread out of the oven. So, we sat on the deck putting gobs of butter on hot slices of bread and washed it down with a glass of ice-cold milk. What a perfect ending to an equine introduction party. In the cool of the evening my wife and I got into my truck and drove home past old dry land wheat fields, and up over Reecer Creek divide past the Dunford Barn. The windows were down and 45 miles an hour seemed more than fast enough. There wasn't much conversation. We looked at each other occasionally and smiled. We were both lost in our thoughts about finding the perfect situation for two old equine gentlemen.

Three or four years later Harriet called to say that when they got up that morning, they found old Arnold lying down quietly in his stall. When they checked further, they realized in fact he had laid down comfortably but permanently and quietly passed on during the night. They said that they were worried about Gazon but he was still eating and seem to be maintaining his usual habits better than expected. Only a few days later they called to say that Gazon too had been found dead that morning. They had a neighbor with a backhoe and he had dug them a large whole up on the hill overlooking the house and barn. The two best friends were placed side by side in the hole and then covered over with four feet of rich loam topsoil. The two had departed this earthly realm during the Indian summer days of early October.

Harriet said, "As I am sure you are well aware, my grumpy old husband George doesn't say too much and doesn't like to display his emotions. But I know I distinctly saw a few tears trickling down his cheeks after the hole was covered. It's not something that we would ever be able to talk about but he does look wistfully up at the hilltop from time to time when he thinks I'm not watching."

Without a job to keep him occupied George didn't last too long either. I noticed his brief obituary in the local newspaper. Their nice yard became overgrown and the barn gradually deteriorated into an unrecoverable state of disrepair. When Harriet died, the land was gobbled up by a nearby developer and a bulldozer quickly erased any evidence that Buck, Gazon, George, and Harriet had ever been there.

Only the memories of those who knew and loved them remained.

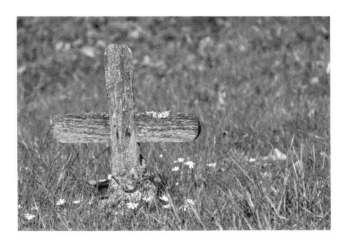

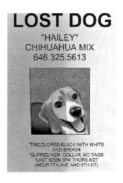

MISSING!

"Have you seen Thor?"

"No! I thought he was with you, when you went up to the property."

"I guess maybe he did. I must have lost track, but he didn't come back with me. I better go back and look and see if he is still there."

Thor was a Keeshond that belonged to a Cle Elum family. Keeshonds are gentle affectionate 35 lb. dogs that develop strong bonds to their two-legged family, especially children. They are descended from Arctic breeds with a double hair coat and are like a smaller version of a Norwegian Elkhound.

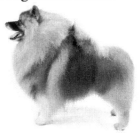

He started out as a silver and black fuzz ball. The undercoat was silver and the guard hairs were tipped with black and it was a little hard to tell which end was which. When one end emitted a playful bold ferocious growl, you knew it was the front end. The other end had a curly handle on it. It didn't take long for him to grow into a playful, inquisitive, loving member of the household and his fearlessness commanded that he be named after one of the Norse Viking gods. Thus, he was christened Thor.

Larry and Nancy had purchased a piece of hillside property on the north side of town and were in the process of cleaning it up so they could build their dream home. The old miner's widow was delighted to unload it when she heard they were interested. They didn't want to steal it from her so they had it appraised and willingly paid her the appraisal amount. The city was renovating, growing, and expanding. There had once been a coal mining era bungalow on the site but it had burned down some years back. It was said to have been the home of her deceased husband's father after he immigrated from Croatia. It was hard dirty work but since it was theirs and they were vested, it was a joy to spend sweat time reclaiming their new property. Thor loved it there too, and when he wasn't supervising Larry and Nancy, he was out patrolling for any varmints or intruders that might dare to set foot in his domain.

Larry hurriedly drove back out and walked the perimeter of the property looking and calling for any sign of his missing assistant. Meanwhile Nancy got on the phone and called all the neighbors to see if anybody had spotted Thor. She also gave us a call at our office as well, asking us to keep our eyes open.

One day passed. Then the second day, and we were now well into the third day. They had put out posters, called all the animal shelters, notified the sheriff's office, groomers, and boarding kennels but there was no response or sign of Thor. They were obviously getting pretty desperate.

"Let's go search the property one last time, " said Nancy. They walked the perimeter and even up into the trees and brush on the steep hillside behind the property. They sat down disconsolately on a stump contemplating their loss before returning home.

" Did you hear that?" said Nancy.

"No!" her husband replied.

"Well, I did! We better go look. It's up there by the old house foundation," said Nancy.

The strange hoarse sound got louder when they approached but they could not determine its origin. Nancy parted some bushes and almost fell into a well concealed hole. The source of the sound was now obvious and they knew it was their long-lost family member. Larry crawled on his hands and knees and peered into the dark hole. Inside was a blessing and a horror all in one. He could just make out silhouette of Thor struggling to stand, neck deep in water at the bottom of an 8-foot deep concrete lined vault. The horrible stench told them that Thor had inadvertently discovered the location of the old house's abandoned septic tank. The ancient rotten wooden lid had collapsed. They found an old broken ladder in the burn pile and used it to climb down into what seemed like the depths of hell. Thor could hardly stand but he wrapped his weak front legs tightly around Larry's neck when lifted out of the hole.

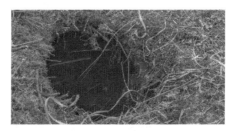

Now it was our turn to help in the rescue. The stench announced their arrival. Fortunately, most of the day's work had been completed and we could dedicate our full efforts Thor's plight.

"Thor had been chasing rats up there. He must have followed one into that jumble," said Larry.

The poor animal was desperately dehydrated in spite of the fact he had been immersed in foul water for three days. His skin was such a mess that the only location to establish an indwelling catheter was in the large jugular vein in his neck. Strong antibiotics and anti-inflammatories were added to the drip. We bathed him in the sink in a solution of a chlorhexidine, and after blow-drying him were able to shave off most of the worst of his ruined haircoat. We had to be extremely careful not to damage the fragile macerated skin underneath. He had obviously been clawing at the concrete walls of the pit trying desperately to get out and had virtually warn his toenails completely off. The pads of his feet were also shredded. After trimming away the worst of the damaged tissue, we cauterized the bleeders and bandaged his feet. Even his front teeth showed signs of unusual wear. Now it was up to Thor.

When Larry and Nancy came to visit, he could barely lift his head and just followed them around the room with his big brown sad eyes. At least he was able to take in some high calorie food processed to the consistency of sloppy mashed potatoes when hand fed by Nancy. Even swallowing was a struggle. There were tears streaming down Nancy's face.

5 days later he tottered out the front door and was gently lifted into the blanketed back of their SUV. He was almost a cartoon caricature of his former self. He must have lost 15 pounds, most of his luxurious hair coat had been shaved or fallen out, and part of his skin was sloughing. He looked like he was wearing astronauts moon landing boots because of the heavily padded bandages on his feet. He soulfully licked Nancy's hand when she reached in to pet him. The only thing that looked promising was the apparent blissful smile on his face and the hint of a sparkle in his eyes.

By that fall he had mostly regained his weight, his skin had cleared up, and he was regrowing beautiful luxurious black and silver haircoat of his Arctic type ancestry.

I said, "It's a good thing he was related to those Norse gods. I don't think there would have been any way he could have survived without all their help."

The next spring, after carefully bulldozing out the old septic tank and house foundation, they began construction of their dream home. Thor could now safely patrol his private empire and keep it free of any dangerous invading varmints.

The house got built and two years later the three of them with a two-legged additional family member came in. Larry said, "I don't think Thor has ever been more than ten feet away from the baby and you need his permission to get closer."

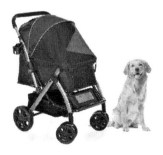

THE END

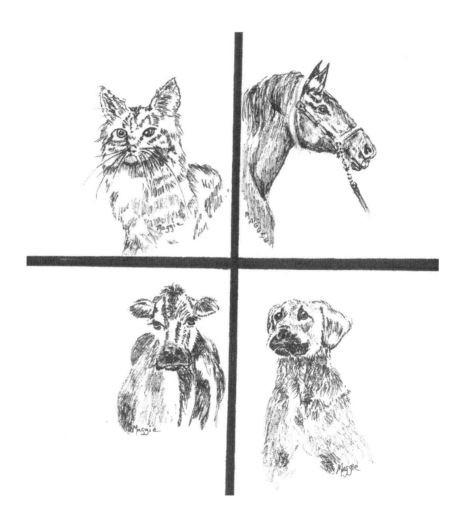

Country Vet

Made in the USA
Lexington, KY
24 November 2019